Dr. Thomas Hoffmann

RITAM

–

The Secret of True Health

Discover the missing element
in medicine and naturopathy

Translated by: Hilary Teske

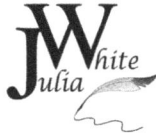

JW Julia White

Disclaimer:
The information and methods presented in this book have been carefully researched and are passed on to the best of our knowledge. Nevertheless neither the author nor the publisher assumes any liability whatsoever for their correct or incorrect application.

The names in the sample cases presented in this book which are not taken from the media have been altered to protect personal privacy.

Julia White Publishing
Internet: www.julia-white.com

ISBN 978-3934402-35-5

Contents

Dedicated to Samuk Deda

–

In deep gratitude

Preface

Dear Reader,

What is health actually? Is one actually healthy when the doctor attests that everything is "okay"? And what if one still feels bad? Are the common degradation and increasing illnesses with advancing age really normal? Are notions of a long, vital life crowned with wisdom and maturity utopian pipe dreams? You will certainly at some time have asked yourself these or similar questions – without finding satisfying answers. In this book you will be led step by step to find the answers within yourself. Together we will set off on a journey of discovery into the secrets of our existence, going far beyond what is understood by "health" today. In doing so, however, you should approach the book free of bias so as to perceive and follow the more extensive details in particular as well. Furthermore, you can understand the book merely as a travelogue or, on top of that, let it inspire you to undertake your own expedition by implementing and trying out some of the recommendations and advice. In that way, you may possibly have your own experiences going far beyond those described here.

At any rate, it is crucial to emphasise that nobody will require you to leave the terrain of reality. On the contrary, the book is supposed to help you experience genuine reality and then yourself judge in how far it is consistent with the usual view of things today. Any changes that take place during this process can only be positive, as the foundation of everything is solely natural laws in this book.

The Author

1. The forgotten instructions for use

Last week Gabriel, a friend we had not seen for a long while, called on us. He looked unwell, overtired, puffy and really at the end of his tether. He immediately started to tell us about his problems without being asked, which was actually unusual for him. He had a problem with his ears, especially the left one, for which doctor had attested 60% loss of hearing. And all that was the result of a terrible bout of flu he had been fighting for four weeks. He felt wretched and simply did not know how to go on. He had been taking the medication prescribed by the doctor for two weeks but it had not helped at all. If there was no improvement by the following week, his doctor wanted to send him to a specialist at the hospital.

My wife offered to press his head a little, which he gladly agreed to. She asked him to lie down on the sofa, knelt down beside his head and began to decongest his lymph with gentle stroking. In doing so, she felt really hard lumps, which also caused pain during the massage. Nevertheless, Gabriel visibly relaxed and when he stood up again he looked much better, much fresher and firmer in the face and his eyes were clear. When he said good-bye, my wife asked him to come by again in the next few days to repeat the lymph drainage. However, he did not do so because he had no time. Besides that, he did not seem to see the need as so pressing any more. One week later, he at any rate reported on the phone that he had been feeling terrific since his visit to us. In the night following it, he had slept fantastically and his hearing was completely normal again. That was clearly the result of the massage, as he had not taken the medicine again since then.

What had happened? Are we witnesses or even perpetrators of a case of miraculous healing? For Gabriel, at any rate, that was what it seemed to be, for we had heard from other friends that he had made comments to them in this regard. This is understandable from his point of view, since, after four long weeks of flu and two endless weeks with greatly restricted hearing, he had experienced not only alleviation but healing within a short time. And that had actually occurred with only a few apparently banal manipulations by my wife, without medication, operations or other lengthy processes, which are otherwise always involved in any healing process in today's medicine. His doctor had not been able to help him either and the medication he had been prescribed had been even less helpful. So was this a prime example of miraculous healing?

The matter looks quite different from our point of view. My wife had not performed a miracle, at least not in the sense of suspending or altering the natural laws. On the complete contrary, she had acted fully in harmony with the laws of nature, by using her hands to help the lymph in Gabriel's head flow freely again. The lymph had become congested because of Gabriel's persistent flu, his wrong behaviour and, additionally, due to the strain from the medication he had taken. Firstly, this severely impeded his natural immune and cleansing reactions and, secondly, impaired his normal mechanisms, such as hearing. Thus, the only correct action was to help remedy the disrupted flow. Everything else then happened quite automatically because of the body's self-healing and self-regenerating mechanisms. Gabriel's good sleep – now possible again without disturbance – the following night did the rest. So we do not have to do with an example of miraculous healing here but rather with an example of correct behaviour towards one's body. Nothing more is indeed necessary, for anyhow only the body can heal itself in the end. No doctor, no medicine, no intervention in the world can heal. The aim always merely consists in supporting the body's self-healing mechanisms, boosting them or removing impediments. If we could manage to keep the body's self-healing mechanisms and its immune system on the highest level without any disruptions, no disease would have the possibility of developing.

So why don't we do that? Because we don't know how it works. And why don't our doctors do it? Because unfortunately they don't seem to know how it works either. We inevitably have to draw this sad or even shocking conclusion from cases like Gabriel's, where a doctor placed an additional strain on the body already weakened by illness by administering drugs, instead of simply bringing relief where there was a blockage with a few hand movements, helping the body to do the rest by itself.

Such examples are unfortunately not uncommon and are also to be found more and more frequently in much more serious and even directly life-threatening diseases. There is now even the medical term "iatrogenic symptoms" for disorders provoked by the doctor, which, according to recent statistics, account for an alarmingly large part of hospital referrals. Apart from a very few exceptions, nobody unfortunately notices this, for we have all lost the knowledge of how our bodies function properly and how they are to be handled correctly.

So we necessarily accept and go along with what the doctors do and prescribe, in the hopeful opinion that they know better about the body's functions on account of their studies. However, the knowledge from their studies is unfortunately confined to a very narrow range of mechanical and chemical functions. They only know extremely little about the global functional structure of our body and mind – and often they do not seem to want to know much more either. For aren't there repeated cases and examples of inexplicable spontaneous healing, even in serious, allegedly incurable cases, which conventional doctors dismiss with lapidary comments? Who has not experienced themselves or heard from others that some old household remedy or seemingly strange alternative method was much more effective and even more successful than conventional medical methods? When such cases occur, when an ulcer can vanish in a very short time without external intervention, when persistent chronic complaints are alleviated and healed almost overnight with a special unusual procedure, shouldn't we get curious as to what mechanisms and processes are at the root of it and try to discover them? If a certain process takes place in one body, it means that it can, in principle, take place in any body. Thus, it would be only logical not to dismiss such "special cases" without understanding but to get to the bottom of them, instead of investing huge sums of research money in projects in which the harmful side-effects almost exceed the positive effects.

A person who follows the repeatedly occurring "inexplicable special cases" with a watchful mind inevitably comes to the conclusion that our body and mind are endowed with an infinitely larger range of functions and mechanisms than we know to date or can even imagine. Here, we want to pursue this track. We want to go on a quest for the lost instructions for use for our body and mind. For we have undoubtedly lost them, as otherwise there would be fewer diseases, disorders and problems, or we could at least cope with them better. Although the notion of instructions for use or a user's manual for our body is certainly somewhat odd at first sight, we still think that we manage quite well with it. After all, we are alive, even live to an increasingly advanced age and have achieved a remarkable level of civilisation. So it can't be all that bad! We will go into more detail on these points later in the book – and experience some surprises.

But first we want to consider an example more familiar to us – the car. With the car everyone knows that instructions for use exist and that following them is crucial for the correct functioning and lifespan of the car, even though most people rely on specialists in car repair shops for this. However, we have to make an important distinction here. There is, in fact, the first part of the instructions, which deals with everyday use, and the second, which describes how to remedy and repair any problems which may arise. Anyone who knows and follows the first part needs to make much less use of the second part. That can be confirmed by all car owners who take care of their cars regularly and make sure that they are correctly used and serviced. They thus save money on repair costs and at the same time increase the lifespan of their vehicles. But all the others also ensure that they do not let the clutch grind, do not drive with the handbrake on and turn off the lights when they get out. For they know – sometimes from bitter experience – that if these basic rules are not adhered to, the car's functioning will be considerably impaired. Every motorist pays the most careful attention to always filling up with petrol in time and exclusively with the proper fuel for their vehicle. For here wrong behaviour has the most direct consequences, namely that you cannot go on driving. With other behavioural disciplinary measures, disregard of which does not have a direct impact, many people are inclined to be sloppier and some of them are not even aware of this. For out of ignorance they do not connect the repeatedly incurring repair costs with their faulty behaviour, e.g. driving with insufficient air pressure in the tyres or not enough oil or cooling water.

In summary, we can retain from this example that it is important to have instructions for use, to know them and follow them in an optimal manner so that, by applying the first part about everyday behaviour correctly, the second part about troubleshooting may become redundant. The second part is only supposed to be used in exceptional cases. In exactly the same way, there must exist instructions for use for our body and mind giving us information on correct everyday behaviour and troubleshooting. For just as there are specific appropriate fuels for the car, there are sure to be appropriate foodstuffs for our body, which promote its functioning, and inappropriate ones, which harm its functioning. Or just as it is important for a car that the oil level is neither too low or too high or that antifreeze is added to the cooling water in winter but not in summer, there are certain to be guidelines for the body as well concerning the quantity and timing of food consumption in general and consumption of specific foodstuffs which are beneficial or harmful to the body's functioning.

From our experience with Gabriel we got to know two examples of behaviours towards the body, one of which complied with the instructions for use and another which did not. The consequence of correct behaviour was "miraculous healing" from Gabriel's subjective point of view. If the knowledge it was based on was part of general knowledge applied by everyone, this would not be anything special but just an absolutely normal case of troubleshooting. If a car which refuses to move from the spot runs again normally after the handbrake has been removed, nobody sees it as a miracle – except perhaps someone who out of ignorance had been looking for the cause of the problem for ages in the wrong place.

What would have happened in Gabriel's case if he had come to us earlier or if he, or at least his doctor, had known the relevant chapter of the instructions for use? Then he would certainly not have had to suffer from loss of hearing for two weeks. The problem with his ear would not have occurred at all if it had been manipulated in time. In that way, his organism would have been spared the side-effects of the medication ordered by the doctor and his psyche – and also his environment – would have been spared the distressing ordeal of his physical impairment. In the case of still earlier manipulation and other correct behavioural elements, his body would probably have dealt with the flu even sooner, or it would only have been a slight cold or not have broken out at all.

We see what a difference it can make if we behave correctly or not and if we only make use of the repair part of the instructions for use or the part on general behaviour as well. For these reasons, it is not only extremely important to find our lost instructions for use again but to make them absolute common knowledge. They should become the major subject in all schools so that nobody is any longer left alone in the most important life issues, namely health and well-being, or dependent on specialists, who, in the end, cannot really help them or only too late.

Now there are naturally considerable differences between our body and a car. Our body is, at any rate, far more complex, is closely connected to our mind and soul and has functions going far beyond mechanical ones. Furthermore, Gabriel's problem was a comparatively harmless case, which would have resolved itself at some point even without a doctor or our help. Can we therefore think globally of instructions for use at all and isn't it utopian to look for such?

There are, however, several counterarguments to these frequently expressed arguments. Firstly, it is the very complexity of our body's structure that makes it much more pressing to handle it properly. For we only have one body and cannot buy a new one repeatedly as with a car. Secondly, our body is an important aid for our mind and the development of our soul, which is why wrong behaviour immediately has more far-reaching repercussions. On the other hand, the unity of body and mind and the innumerable intelligent structures and cycles in our body make it almost imperative for it to be based on a structure set out in a manual of correct behaviour, also making it much less complicated than one might at first think. After all, the allegedly so harmless cases, as in our initial example, are the very ones which impair our well-being and functioning the most and longest, and – if repeated and accumulated over a long period – lead to serious permanent damage. For that reason, it would be desirable and worthwhile to have an appropriate guide to behaviour precisely for such "harmless little things."

As we will see later in this book, there are many indications in ourselves, in nature and in old written records suggesting that it is anything but utopian to look for instructions for use for our body and mind. These indications show, however, that we have not only forgotten how we should handle our bodies and minds properly but also what functions and mechanisms they are endowed with at all.

That can best be illustrated by extending our example of the car. Let's imagine we are in a country or a civilisation where cars are unknown. One day the inhabitants are given a car, but without instructions and with an empty tank. The people now naturally start to examine the mysterious gift attentively and try it out. After a while, they find out that they can open the doors and make themselves comfortable inside and that they can produce light and a shrill sound with it. Then one of the experimenters turns the ignition key and as the car is in gear, it jolts forward. Once the first shock is over, everyone is thrilled and they now understand that they can transport themselves in this machine. As long as you turn the key and hold it, you can move forward in jolts. What a wonderful thing!

The next difficulties can, of course, be foreseen as soon as the battery gives up the ghost. But before that happens, the experimenters have noticed that the forward movement must have something to do with the special box under the car bonnet. For if they disconnect one of the cables in it, the whole thing ceases to work. As they are familiar with electricity, they soon have the battery problem under control and they thus use the machine they have been given as a means of transportation, especially to transport heavy objects.

Then one day comes a stranger, who has observed their use of the car and after a while calls the team leader to come to him. He wants to confide a secret to him, with which they can awaken quite different, downright incredible powers in their machine. The team leader shows interest and so the stranger tells him about the correct functioning and handling of the car. Although it all sounds rather complicated, they still want to try it. So the team leader has the tank filled with fuel, sits down at the wheel himself, presses the clutch and turns the ignition key. Nothing happens! Although the familiar noise is heard, the car does not move forward as before. He tries again, this time somewhat longer. Suddenly the car starts to drone, wobble and smoke. In alarm, he lets go the clutch and the car shoots forward like a rocket. The stranger was right. These mysterious procedures have provoked such an escalation of the car's way of functioning that there is no comparison with what they had known before. We can justifiably speak of a quantum leap.

But let's return to our subject of true health. What does the little story have to do with us? Might it be possible that we, too, have not only lost the instructions for use for our body and mind but also the awareness of their real function mechanisms? That's impossible! Or have we? Didn't Einstein claim we used only 5 – 10% of our brain's potential? Don't medical experts and biologists who research our brain say that the task and function of the largest part of it have not yet been explained? Don't modern genetic researchers consider more than 90% of our DNA, i.e. our genes, to be unimportant – or at least unintelligible – data waste? Aren't there organs, such as the tonsils or appendix, which modern health professionals consider to be functionless and meaningless, thus even removing them prophylactically in an operation? Don't we often hear of people with special exceptional or even supernatural abilities? Might it be that these abilities are just as little paranormal as the correctly handled car in the story above? If that was the case, we would in our present existence perhaps be so far away from the real, normal human existence as the jolting car was from its function as a vehicle. Then, in all that contemporary scientists declare to be unexplained, unexplored, unintelligible or meaningless lies the potential for a quantum leap into the unimaginable. And if that is the case, all of us – the population, medical doctors and naturopaths

– do not have the faintest clue as to what real health actually means.

Can that be possible? Let's listen to ourselves, examine what we feel, taking seriously all our present or previous inklings that life is supposed to be something different from what we are experiencing today.

But no matter what your answer looks like now, join us on our adventuresome journey to discover the secret of true health. That will be the most interesting and worthwhile journey you can ever make, and at the end you yourself – and not the book – will give the answer.

2. Friend or foe?

"Impossible!" a lady of resolute appearance piped up. "Completely impossible! I am a business woman, you know! I have a shop and I simply can't schedule my time like that."

I was in the music room of a village school in the Swiss Alps, where I was giving a presentation on Ritam Samation to an audience of about 20. I had explained the technique and particularly the purpose of Samation in detail, had gone into the difference between Samation and meditation and was just explaining what the whole thing looked like in everyday life. I emphasised that the crucial thing was to practise Ritam Samation regularly and continually twice a day for about 30 minutes.

Upon these words the lady – let's call her Elli – interrupted me. She was sitting at the front on the right, must have been in her mid-forties, was a little plump and radiated great dynamism and resoluteness. She looked around the room and saw some people nodding in agreement. I calmly replied to her comment:

"Nothing is impossible. It's only a question of whether we want it or not. We manage to find enough time for so many things under the most difficult conditions if we only want to! What a lot of time we spend every day in front of the TV or newspaper, in the end just to burden our consciousness with trivialities or nonsense! We all have our free will. So I don't want to and won't force or persuade you to do anything. I only want to give you information as a basis for you to then make a decision of your own free will. It's up to you how you decide. But you should also be clear about what you want in life. For although you have your absolutely free will, which nobody can take away, you then have to bear the consequences of your free decision. Nobody can relieve you of this responsibility either. And for this it is good to have information and become clear about things.

If you care about your health – true health –you have to do something for it. Nothing comes from nothing. And after all the mistakes we have made in the past concerning our bodies and minds – and we always had time for those mistakes, too –, we should begin as soon as possible to go in a different direction. You can't expect what you have accumulated gradually over many years to suddenly disappear overnight. In spite of all its miraculous effects, Ritam Samation isn't a miraculous technique that makes good everything we have botched up through our behaviour again with a snap of the fingers."

After that, I repeated the technical details, announced the date for the beginning of the course and concluded my presentation.

The course started two days later and Elli was one of the participants. She had thought about her priorities and at least wanted to give it a try. The following day she came to me for a Darshana, a one-to-one counselling session, and told me about her digestive and weight problems. She had already tried all possible slimming and other diets but her excess kilos were simply stubborn. Besides that, she often struggled with flatulence, above all when she ate more fresh food. Her digestion also left much to be desired. She had bowel movements only two or three times a week and sometimes even less often. What was the correct diet for her? Or should she go on a fast?

The essence of the advice I gave her in that Darshana can be summarised in two pieces of old popular wisdom:

1. Only eat when you are really hungry and stop eating when it tastes best.

2. You should drink your food and eat your drink.

The second rule means you should chew and insalivate the food so well that it becomes liquid before you swallow it and that you should also insalivate drinks well, meaning actually "chew" them. In reality, I also gave her a third piece of advice. But I would like to go into that at a later point in the book.

After a week I saw Elli again and she told me proudly and full of joy that she had already lost 3 kg and had bowel movements once or twice a day. The day before, it had even been three times.

That again was one indication why a young woman from the south of Germany came to the Darshana with her two-year-old son a couple of months ago. She told me that she had spent two weeks with friends in the east of Turkey. It had been awful there, as there had been nothing to eat besides bread, yoghurt, some vegetables from the garden and water. Her children had complained of constant hunger. And since the trip her youngest son had filled his nappy regularly three times a day. She had to change his nappies after every meal. She was afraid that he had got an intestinal infection and her paediatrician had also asked her to come again if nothing changed within the next few weeks. After I had made certain that it was not a question of diarrhoea and that the consistency of the stool was quite normal, I asked:

"Were you able to observe what the other children there in Turkey ate and what their bowel movements were like?"

"None of them have much to eat and some of them get up from the table hungry. And now you mention it, I remember. They all had to go to the toilet so often or at least the little ones, where you could notice it!"

At any rate, I congratulated her on her son's digestion and urged her to make sure it stayed like that, according to the rule: As often as we eat a day, as often must bowel movements take place. When she looked at me rather puzzled, I explained the connection to her. Join us on this little excursion into our digestive system. We will meet Elli again later.

People in the poorer regions of eastern Turkey, about whom we have just been speaking, live – as far as diet is concerned – as most people did a few hundred years ago or like animals in the wild. None of them think of eating at all until they are hungry. They do not live in an affluent society like ours, where eating has become a pastime and a social event and it is not hunger which determines if and when we eat, but appetite, boredom, social occasions, the striking of the clock and snacks between meals which smell enticing or stimulate the appetite. With all that, hunger has been forgotten and is actually fought like an enemy. We, thus, pay scrupulous attention to always having something edible at hand in case our stomach begins to rumble. Viewed physiologically, however, that is totally wrong, as hunger is anything but an enemy. We can see that best in wild animals or primitive peoples, who do not think about eating until they are hungry and only then go in search of food, which requires a high degree of energy, stamina and sharpness of the senses. With predators, for example, it may take several days for them to track down a prey, which they then have to kill. And they do all that in a state of ravenous hunger! Once they have eaten, their energy and sharpness of the senses are at an end. A fully satiated lion, for example, sleeps up to 24 hours at a stretch.

Hence, hunger is far more than just a signal indicating that the body desires food. In fact, it also prepares the digestive system for the next intake of food by initiating the coating of the large and small intestines with mucous, thus provoking defaecation. At the same time, it mobilises power and energy in the body, putting the mind and senses completely on the alert. In addition, in a state of ravenous hunger the digestive system is able to obtain everything optimally from the food and metabolise what the body needs. Let's imagine our digestion is a fire which blazes so fiercely with "burning" hunger that it can really burn everything, even not so good or overabundant food. In this state, our metabolism even catabolises waste products and harmful substances in our whole body which would otherwise be detrimental to our health. However, if the fire only glows faintly and is about to go out, only smoke and fumes emerge from even the best fuel, i.e. the best, purest, most organic, wholest of foods, all the more so when they are consumed in too large a quantity. That is the mistake that almost all nutritional systems and theories make. They concentrate solely on the "what" but forget the "how." But what is the use of all the precious – and often expensive – vegetarian, macrobiotic, alkaline-acid balanced, specially combined, whole, energetic light food if the digestive system is not prepared for it at all nor able to utilise it correctly?

Therefore hunger is the key to correct and healthy eating. If you eat with real hunger, your food is optimally and completely digested and all its contents are made use of. At the same time, all our senses are so alert and sharp that they again serve as reliable signposts to our proper food. In our current state of dullness, in their degeneration they unfortunately all too often cheat us with the good taste or scent of those very foodstuffs which are unhealthy or harmful. As hunger also stimulates the bowel to cleanse and empty itself, it automatically puts an end to any constipation problems, resulting in the natural rhythm, in which a bowel movement occurs at the latest shortly after each intake of food. Only in this way is congestion avoided in the digestive system. Through his holiday in Turkey without sweets and snacks between meals, the little boy had found a natural rhythm in harmony with the laws of the digestive system, in which there is a bowel movement as often a day as someone has had a meal, contrary to all the prophecies of doom by alleged experts, who themselves eat wrongly.

If we consider all these points, the question arises as to why we actually view hunger as an enemy. Isn't it rather one of our best friends, bringing us so many boons beneficial to our health? As so often, the answer lies in our ignorance, in the fact that we have forgotten the instructions for use. However, all Earth's cultures had their rise and heyday under Spartan conditions, where hunger was the order of the day. When people "at last did not have to suffer hunger anymore" and affluence set in, a decline always started. Today also we, who virtually keep ourselves continually in the state of the satiated lion out of fear of hunger, rather provide a prime example of degeneration than a shining example of the crown of creation. The roots of this schizophrenia are already to be found some generations previously. For although in every period of hardship people personally experienced what vitality and fitness they had in such situations and although the nobility in their affluence had always provided an exact counterexample with their ailments and degeneration, the wish became deeply rooted in "common people" to be able to "live the life of Riley" like the nobility. Today, this wish has been fulfilled and we are just as sick and degenerate as the nobility has always been. In this regrettable state, we are naturally glad of any relief or help, even if it is not any real help, and use all the little remedies and powders which doctors provide - uncontrolledly and thoughtlessly without wanting to recognise or accept that these only spiral us further into the vicious circle. So on a closer look, our supposed friends turn out to be enemies and our alleged enemy a friend.

This is the point at which we should wake up, become aware of the current state of affairs and set priorities. If these priorities are other than to go on letting ourselves drift until our passing, we also have to take appropriate action. And the first, most important – and fortunately the easiest – action consists in recultivating hunger. For this we do not need to starve or go on a special fast. We simply fast three times a day by waiting so long with each intake of food until we feel hunger and then "enjoy" it for a good half-hour. After the remarks above, you can perhaps to some degree imagine what a profound impact this simple act has on our well-being and our health. However, you cannot really comprehend it until you have tried it, and not only for a few days but for at least six months. For things do not go as quickly and easily for everyone as they did for Elli. But after six months everyone can judge from their own experience whether it is the right thing or not.

Naturally, many people will have doubts or counterarguments. Housewives, in particular, will in alarm imagine their family members all coming hungry at different times and wanting to eat. However, even if that were the case, the question must be permitted as to what is more important – a regulated eating rhythm or a healthy family. But fortunately the natural laws also come to our aid here. For if you eat when you are really hungry and stop eating when the food tastes best, your next hunger will come in about five hours, as experience shows. This is regardless of whether you do physical or mental work, if you are fat or thin, old or young. This rhythm, which of course will not start immediately on the first day, will thus become the basis for a new eating schedule in the family after a while, but then consistent with the eating rhythm of each individual member of the family.

In other words, you can plan your eating behaviour in advance. If the lunch break in your firm does not allow flexible eating times, you just adjust the size and time of your breakfast so that your hunger comes half an hour at the latest before your lunch break. The same applies for invitations, business or celebration meals or other unavoidable eating appointments.

Doesn't that already look like the first elements of instructions for use? And isn't it far simpler than expected? The reason is that we only have to bother about our behaviour as our body's intelligence takes over the rest. In the chapter after next we will recognise in greater depth how wonderful it is and how even the smallest processes interact in an incredible manner.

But let's return to the correct behaviour concerning food. The first basic rule in this respect said that we should only eat when we are really hungry. However,for this we must first get to know what hunger is again. For who of the post-war generation has really experienced hunger? The "ravenous hunger" which is meant here is, in fact, considerably different from appetite, which we today commonly confuse with hunger. For example, our appetite quickly disappears when we imagine we only have dry bread to eat or when we drink a glass of water. In contrast, real hunger is not influenced by anything like that. In this state, we would eat anything we can get our teeth into. Neither does a rumbling stomach always have to do with hunger. In general, we can say that if we wonder whether we are hungry, we certainly do not have hunger at that moment. For true hunger – ravenous hunger – is beyond all doubt. It is an absolutely characteristic feeling, which we will not forget so quickly. Therefore it suffices to practise a few times and gain experience, for example by going for a walk or a hike without having had breakfast until the unmistakable feeling of hunger comes after five hours at the latest.

Above all, we should also lose our fear of it and quite calmly permit it, observe it and get a feel for it. We will not starve or lose weight that quickly and a fear of this is not justified. However, we will have a new experience, get to know a previously unknown aspect of our body and realise that there is actually nothing hostile about it. Everything else was and is only an acquired figment of our imagination. In reality, only a very few people who starved to death really died of hunger. Most of them died from their fear and illusions or were poisoned by their own toxins, which released themselves from their gut due to their long abstention from food. Isn't it a paradox that one person dies after a few weeks without food while another voluntarily goes without food for 30 or 40 days to cleanse themselves and in the hope of becoming enlightened? Why doesn't the second person die, too, or why doesn't the first make progress towards enlightenment? It is because they have programmed thrmselves differently. So let's change our hunger programming. It is completely safe to admit hunger for half an hour before each meal. From time to time, we can even plan a day of fasting when we only drink water. Death from starvation does not threaten until hunger of the tissue occurs after four or five weeks without food and which normally nobody can voluntarily ignore. Everything else is completely harmless but will provide us with new experience concerning our body – and our mind! – and also do a great service to our health. However, we should only undertake long fasts under expert instruction and supervision and not until we have prepared our body for them at least for a year with proper behaviour towards food.

Once we have got to know and appreciate hunger again, we come to the second basic rule of food intake, namely stopping eating when your food tastes best. That is so important because we should not completely fill our stomach so that digestion has sufficient room to function optimally. Otherwise the stomach has to extend itself or push undigested food back into the oesophagus, which we experience as acid reflux. In general, about one quarter of the stomach should be empty after eating and that is almost exactly achieved when the food tastes best. At the beginning, it will probably not be easy for you to catch the right moment in time. But our instructions for use can also help us again here. If we have to wait more than five hours before we feel hungry again, we have eaten too much. However, if we feel hungry much earlier, we ate too little. In this way, we can return to the correct perception and behaviour by observing our feeling of hunger.

In addition, the rule of chewing and insalivating our food thoroughly will be another valuable help. For one of the greatest problems with eating is the speed of it. Most people today eat so quickly that they have already overfilled their stomachs in the time the stomach needs to signal the feeling of saturation to our consciousness. However, that cannot happen if we chew our food thoroughly and with enjoyment. Then the impulses of the digestive system can be implemented in time and the stomach gets overfilled much less often.

Chewing is, of course, also important for another reason. For the food can only be optimally metabolised if it has been ground up into fine enough pieces. Besides that, it has to be mixed as well as possible with saliva, which as well as having a pre-digestive function above all effects the transmission of information to the digestive system, which is crucial for the further correct processes. None of these processes can take place when we just gulp down our food – and drink as well –, in the belief that the stomach will manage. If that was the case, we would not need any saliva or molar teeth. And if we did not need them, we would not have them either.

We have thus come to the end of the first important chapter of the instructions for use for our body and have now also understood why Elli had such rapid success "only" through following this simple advice. Everyone can – and should – now start implementing it immediately so as get his own personal experiences. Otherwise everything will remain pure theory, which you simply accept or reject.

For real change, however, you need your own experience for yourself. In the next chapter we will see what such experience can look like in the long term.

3. The myth of eternal life

Immortality! An age-old human dream. In all cultures and at all times, there have been mythological reports of people who attempted to fathom the secret of eternal life, of saints or "sons of God" who lived a very long time on earth, of fountains of youth and mysterious rejuvenation cures giving people back their youthful freshness and helping them live longer. In today's age of rationality, such reports are, at best, viewed as entertaining sagas or fairy tales with a psychological interpretation. But the myth of eternal life still has its place in our heads and hearts today as well. However, it is mostly no longer related to the body but has been shifted to other levels. In the past centuries, at least religions and spirituality were able to provide most people with the prospect of an existence beyond their very limited time on Earth. But these dimensions are today taken less and less seriously, which is why recent scientific theories have shifted the discussion about longevity to our genes. According to this, the purpose of our life on Earth consists in helping our genes to attain the maximal survival success. Those who have as many children and grandchildren as possible preserve their genes in the next generations, thus ensuring their "life after death." For many people that is not enough or too impersonal so that they "immortalise" themselves through political action, in the worst case through wars or dictatorships. Others eternalise themselves through scientific or artistic works or financial investments, which are supposed to outlast time in the form of foundations or humanitarian organisations. In recent times even ordinary people who cannot make themselves a name politically, scientifically or artistically –let alone financially – have the possibility of being remembered after their death due to some exceptional – however absurd – unique feat in the Guinness Book of Records.

However, for a few people that is all too abstract as well and so they place their unlimited trust in science and technology, namely that of the future. They have their bodies – sometimes only their heads – frozen after their death, in the hope that human advances in future decades or centuries will allow them to reawaken their frozen corpses to new – more everlasting – life. Where does this deep human longing to live long or even eternally come from? Is it only a figment of our imagination or does it have a serious foundation? Everyone has certainly at some time or other thought about the strange time distribution that normally characterises a human life today. After an unusually long childhood, in which we are more or less strongly dependent on our parents' care, we only begin to stand on our own feet in life after about two decades. Then follows the phase in which we search for and find our place in life, during which we are physically and mentally in top form. But, astonishingly, this phase is shorter than the first phase of development. Most experts concur that our physical decline already begins between 28 and 35 and even proceeds quite rapidly in some people. Our mental capacity generally remains a few years longer but then also starts to decline. Our strength decreases, we are less fit, the first aches and pains appear and illnesses become our constant companions. We are getting old. After the age of 40 everyone makes regular visits to the doctor, every 50-year-old has at least one operation behind them, after 60 we start to get dependent again, on the nursing care of others, and eventually die. That seems to be the sad reality everyone experiences personally and much more in the examples of friends and relatives and indeed of the whole of humanity. And some people still do not want to simply accept it. And they are right! For alone the process of slow decline and decay is an unusual process in nature. All living beings in in the wild – fauna and flora – grow, thrive and constantly develop throughout their lives up to the moment when they die – possibly after a short phase of decline. No tree, no wolf or antelope declines like a human being for over half its life. So why does a human as the crown of creation?

There is another question mark if we relate the human lifespan, particularly the phase of full physical and mental capacity to the growing, developing and learning phase of childhood. Isn't it a downright waste of energy of nature to let a person grow up into what defines a human being under the close care of their parents for 20 years, only to abandon them to decline and decay after another 10 – 15 years and, in the end, let them die in a mostly wretched physical and mental state after some years of infirmity and need of nursing care, the extent of which often surpasses that of infancy? Nowhere is a similar relation to be found in the animal world in the wild. Although there are in fact many animals that have a shorter lifespan, they also have a comparatively much shorter phase of childhood and development. The relation is always quite different, more productive and more meaningful. So the question again arises: Why is the human, the crown of creation, so negatively out of line?

Scientific research unfortunately does not provide an answer to this question. For it actually starts with the existing "normal case," analyses it statistically and at most describes the underlying processes as normal and unalterable reality. Only a very few – probably the "greater minds" – seem to see outside the box of normality and think profoundly about it. The well-known doctor and stress researcher Dr. Hans Selye writes: "In all my autopsies (and I have carried out over 1000) I have never seen a person who died of old age. In general, I don't think a single person has ever died of old age. We inevitably die because a vital part of our body has worn out prematurely in relation to the rest."

Doesn't that remind us of our comparison to the car? Only a very few good cars actually break down because of faulty construction or wrong assembly, but it happens because vital parts give up the ghost due to wrong use or insufficient maintenance. That all too often begins with failure to change the oil, a too low level of oil, dirty filters or similar "trivialities."

But here we come up against the limit of our comparison. For when a mechanical fault has occurred in a car – whether through incorrect handling or an accident – a repair is unavoidable. Even if you instead start looking after and servicing it in absolute compliance with every single section of the instructions for use, the damage cannot be remedied by itself and will mostly even get worse until the car is irreparably broken. However, it is different with our bodies. The body is equipped with sophisticated self-repairing mechanisms, which normally keep all parts and functions in perfect condition if we don't throw a spanner in the works. These mechanisms even go far beyond the mere repair and correction of damage. Thus, our body is in fact continually occupied with a constant complex process of renewing all its parts – atom by atom. In this way, it ensures in an extremely intelligent manner that the more sensitive and more worn tissue is replaced in a rapid rhythm and the more robust and less heavily stressed tissue somewhat more slowly, thus making everything continually available in a new, unused form. After about a year, almost all the atoms in our body have been replaced by new ones – an absolutely inconceivable procedure. For that reason, there should be no problems or disorders at all due to wear and tear or degeneration.

To illustrate this, let's imagine we live in a house in which all the parts were replaced every year brick by brick. An invisible power would be constantly occupied with taking out one brick after another and carefully replacing it with a new one until the whole house consisted of new building elements, while still retaining its old form. In such a house we would never have to worry about wear and tear, let alone disintegration. Even damage occurring at one time due to external influences would not be permanent. After a year at the latest, it would have disappeared again in the course of the automatic process of renewal. Isn't that a fantastic notion? However, the fact that we actually live in such a house – our body – is far more fantastic. For today our body is no longer the same as it was a year ago, every one of its atoms has been replaced by a new one in the meanwhile. And in one year it will not be the same as it is today. Every minute particle will then be new, renewed, replaced. Hence, any disorders, any degeneration, wear and tear and even impairments due to our disfigured environment will also have vanished by then!

But stop! There seems to be an error somewhere. For we do have diseases, problems and damage which we also had last year and two years ago. And they do not seem to have got better but rather worse and worse. There must be a mistake somewhere. But where? We can certainly trust the scientists who have proved that this replacement process takes place, for they are very good at making such series of quantitative measurements. And it would not be crucial either even if they had erred by a few months concerning the duration of the whole process. So we have to look elsewhere.

Based on our comparison with the house we can actually only imagine three possible causes of this paradox:

1. The whole replacement process is wrongly or improperly controlled. If, for example, single parts of the house are omitted by mistake or the replacement process is carried out in such a way that cracks in the wall are not repaired but carefully preserved, the house would naturally not be "new" after one year.

2. The new raw material used to replace the old is faulty. Then there would not be any improvement but possibly even a deterioration of the present state if, for example, a porous brick was replaced by a faulty or even more porous one or if certain building elements were simply missing and could not be renewed.

3. The damage occurs more quickly than the repairs. If, for example, a window is shattered every week but only one is replaced every four weeks, the renewal process has no chance of keeping pace. It is exactly the same when a hole in the roof becomes bigger with every gust of wind and every rainfall, affecting other parts of the house.

What does all that mean in relation to our body?

The third case is clear. If we have a bad accident or have a really acute and life-threatening illness, it is insane to trust the annual process of renewal and not take immediate emergency measures. But we have not spoken of such cases here either.

The second case obviously relates to our nutrition. We are more likely to find the answer here. For it is quite obvious that the result of the renewal of our body can only be as good as the raw materials available. If we predominantly feed our body with inferior foodstuffs, which possibly do not contain some of the essential substances at all, we cannot expect the process of replacement to result in a complete renewal. In this point, we do not need to search long to find indications, examples and recommendations – from conventional medicine as well – showing that the usual diet today plays a big role in most degenerative diseases. We eat too much fat, too much protein, too much sugar, too little fibre, too few vitamins and minerals, just to name a few examples. In addition, the ingredients are influenced and altered again through industrial manufacturing and processing and through the preparation and combination with other foodstuffs. Here we are speaking exclusively of the substances and molecules constituing our food without considering its information content. We will go into more detail about the latter in a later chapter.

As if our own experiences were not already bad enough, experiments have also been carried out on innocent rats concerning this matter. We still do want to mention these since they might provide additional insight for someone or other. Various groups of laboratory rats were each given the typical diet of a specific society under otherwise identical conditions. At an age corresponding to 50 in a human being, the rats were killed and an autopsy carried out. The result showed that each group displayed the very same diseases to be found in the equivalent human society. Thus, for example, the rats with a typical British diet showed the same incidence of heart disease, cancer, diabetes, etc. as the British population. Even for the most unaccepting person that ought to be sufficient proof that today's customary fast food, industrially produced convenience food and other bad habits which have entered our own kitchens are more than detrimental to our health and life expectancy.

But there are also people who have recognised that and are trying to eat more consciously by incorporating more fruit, vegetables and fresh food into their diets but still do not have the indestructible, eternally youthful health which actually should be the result of the process of renewal. What is the reason for that? Part of the problem, which does not however only affect these people, lies in our foodstuffs themselves. Thus, extensive investigations of ingredients show, for example, that a cauliflower or a carrot bought today only contains a fraction of the minerals the same vegetable had 30 or 40 years ago. Even if you consciously eat a healthy diet, your body no longer finds the substances which are actually to be expected. The cause lies in our modern industrial and chemical agriculture, which has depleted the soil so much that a major part of the vegetables in the supermarket is actually only artificial fertilizer saved from decay by pesticides and packed in a colorful wrapping. Organic farming certainly provides an alternative here, as it ensures a much more natural growth of plants. However, especially because of the high prices, we have to check exactly if what is written on the outside is actually contained inside. For not every instance of "controlled farming" is organic. Another problem arises mostly with organic fruit. On account of the high prices and the still often inadequate storage and transport facilities in the health food shops, wastage is a significant economic factor. Therefore fruits are often harvested in an even less ripe state than in conventional commerce so that the valuable natural substances cannot form at all. The end result is an apple or tomato which was indeed able to grow in a very natural way but was finally harvested before it had developed all the substances so important for our health.

An increasing number of people see so-called nutritional supplements as a way out of this problem. Those are products, mostly in tablet form, which are supposed to contain all that is missing from our food. The basic idea of this approach is certainly not unreasonable. It goes back to the twice Nobel prize winner Linus Pauling, who had already occupied himself with the necessary raw materials for our metabolism at the beginning of the 1970's. He was particularly interested in vitamin C and carried out an experiment on himself to prove that the regular intake of vitamin C increases life expectancy.

When he died at the age of 93 in 1994, it seemed that he had managed to prove this. However, he also claimed that vitamin C was a
prophylaxis against cancer and still got prostate cancer in 1991. Like
most people today, he did not realise – and as a representative of our
modern scientific system perhaps was not able to recognise at all –
that no isolated substances exist either in the human body or in living
nature. Everything is an interaction, a connection, a combination of
the various elements, which only achieve their effect in this specific
connection and combination. Single isolated components are therefore much less effective or even not at all.

We have thus finally come to the perhaps most important point as
far as our food is concerned, namely our metabolism. In the previous
few pages we spoke a lot about ingredients, their necessity for our
body and their presence in food. But what use are all these ingredients
even in an infinite quantity if our digestive system has lost the ability
to extract them from the food? We then eat healthy food, expensive
organic vegetables, even more expensive supplements and simply ex-
crete them – more or less unprocessed – with our next bowel movement. But our body is still lacking the badly needed raw materials. This
is the point where we should begin, for if our metabolism does not
function we do not need to think about one or another substance in
our food. But aren't we caught in a hopeless vicious circle there? For
how can we ever extract the necessary substances which our metabolism needs to become healthy again from our food without a healthy
metabolism? But don't worry! Here it is not a problem of too little
but of too much. In order to make our digestive fire, which we spoke
about in the previous chapter, blaze brightly again, we do not in fact
have to give it some additional substances but we have to relieve it. For
the problem of our digestive system just described corresponds to the
situation when the fire is only still glowing dimly, is almost going out
and then has a mountain of fuel piled on it. Only if we relieve it, will
it stop fuming and smoking and regain strength. Our digestive system
has lost its strength through years of overloading and improper strain.
Let's just remember that the actual normal state is an empty stomach
and empty intestines, which mobilise their powers for a brief time
after an intake of food, process the food and then return to a state of
rest. In contrast, most people's current reality is a constantly full and
stressed stomach, which we often do not even allow to rest at night.
Countless little snacks, nibbling, sampling, here a morsel, there a bite
mean that our digestive system is in a state of constant stress – often

not exactly with easily digestible substances. In addition, there are the many mutually incompatible foods which we mix or eat together. Thus our stomach and our intestines have to juggle constantly and cannot bring any digestive work to an end because new unsolicited and mostly inappropriate things are continually arriving. Is it a wonder that their performance increasingly declines over time? And we have not even spoken of mental strains due to stress in this connection.

The only solution lies in our new friend from the previous chapter - hunger. We must consistently and regularly cultivate proper hunger again, thus making our digestive fire blaze as fiercely as possible so that the subsequent food is optimally and completely digested, processed and metabolised. Then the problem of the raw materials required is solved almost automatically. For the important raw materials our body needs to carry out its processes of repair and renewal are still contained in healthy, varied, natural food in sufficient quantities.

Concerning this, there is also a very interesting experiment which was conducted by the Massachusetts Institute of Technology (MIT). A group of mice was given 40% less to eat than a normally fed control group (measured by the number of calories). The result was that their life expectancy doubled! Shouldn't that give us food for thought and make hunger even more appealing to us?

To emphasise it once again, it does not mean starving. It is only a matter of making hunger a regular part of our everyday behaviour. In return, we will be rewarded with better health and greater longevity.

"But what sort of life is that! If I'm not allowed to have any pleasures anymore, I'd rather do without the few extra years!" I often hear such objections in lectures or counselling when we get to speak of this topic. But unfortunately this is a great and downright tragic misunderstanding. For the constant satiation and overeating most of us live with at the moment does not only lead to more diseases and to greater degeneration. Above all, it makes us dull physically and mentally, deprives us of joy in life, vitality, lightness and even those very pleasures of the senses which are the reason for us actually doing all that. Our senses of taste and smell become so blunted that they require greater and greater stimulation to be able to perceive anything at all. We can hardly speak of proper pleasure at all anymore! In contrast, anyone who cultivates their hunger again will experience how their senses become sharper, how they can increasingly perceive finer scents and tastes, how food which they had disparagingly compared to polystyrene and cardboard not so long ago suddenly tastes good. Only then do we get to know fine tastes, delicate scents and real pleasure again, not only in connection with food. For with the proper way of eating the whole body becomes more sensitive and everybody can wait with interest to see what physical and also sexual peak experiences are in store for them, when they lead their body to them through correct behaviour. In brief, the pleasures and joys of life do not become fewer when we cultivate hunger but exactly the contrary happens: only then do we get to know true enjoyment, which we are currently chasing after convulsively, but in vain.

Concerning this subject, I would like to tell you about a woman who was in all the media in the 1970's. She was called Eula, 81 years old, 160 cm tall and had had her standard weight of 45 kg for 40 years. She suffered from high blood pressure, heart problems and arthritis. However, her main problem was intermittent peripheral artery occlusive disease (nicknamed "shop window disease" in German). She could only walk about 30 m at the most before she was smitten with such severe pain in her calves that she had to stop – mostly in front of a shop window to conceal her problem. Her pain was often even so unrelenting that she had to be carried home. The reason was circulatory disorders in her legs caused by arteriosclerosis, deposits in her blood vessels. She also had the same problem in her hands and it was so severe that she had to wear gloves in summer. Furthermore, she had been suffering from angina pectoris for 15 years and had been hospitalised five years before because of a heart attack. At the age of 81 she heard of a system which was said to cure cardiovascular disease and even arthritis through a change of diet and light, strengthening, dynamic exercise. She informed herself, changed her diet and started on the programme. Four years later – Eula was then 85 – she was so well again that she took part in the Olympic Games for seniors and won the gold medal in both the half-mile and one-mile running races. She took part again a year later and won two gold medals again. At the age of 90 she still ran a mile every day.

This case shows us in an impressive way that our body's natural repair and regeneration mechanisms are able to renew the body enduringly even in very advanced diseases and at a great age – when we give them the proper conditions. Our diet plays the most important and fundamental role in this but proper exercise is also of great importance.

However, we can see something else from this example. And now we come back to the first point in our previous reflections, where we wondered if perhaps the whole bodily exchange process might be functioning in a faulty manner and be incorrectly controlled. For who actually controls this process? Our mind does. Besides all the physical factors we have already spoken about, the mind plays a crucial role. For it influences not only our behaviour, which is, in the end, also indirectly responsible for our bodily functions, but directly and indirectly controls the constant renewal of our body as well. If our mind erroneously believes a "crack in the wall" to be normal, it will control the replacement of the bricks in such a way that the crack is actually preserved and does not disappear; or if it considers some damage to be irremediable, it will not effect any renewal.

With all her infirmities, Eula could have said that after all she was 81 and therefore not in a worse state than the average American. Most of her fellows and even the doctors would probably have confirmed that, as at that age it is actually normal to have already died. If you are still alive, diseases of old age are, at any rate, the order of the day. If she had thought like that, her mind would also have passed on that reality to her body, for it would also have been her reality. Then she would have lived for a while getting along with her problems more or less well and died – a completely normal case. But Eula did not think like that. Something in herself had made her believe that even at her age and with her diseases an improvement must be possible and led her to go on a search for it. She thus started to give her body a different foundation on a material level through her diet and exercise and on a mental level through her attitude. We have seen the result.

The question arising from this is: What is actually "normal"? This question goes far beyond being purely scientific or philosophical. For by the answer we give we shape our own fate, our own future. Nevertheless, every person must answer this question for themselves, even though they can very well orient themselves by the large majority – or by the few who show by their example that something different is possible and the state of the majority in reality only represents a regrettable error. If someone like Eula is capable of making such a turnaround at the age of 81, as in the now hundreds and thousands of documented cases, it should be clear to us that degeneration after the age of 28 – 35 is not an error of nature but a human error. Then we know where the undefinable longing for a long life in health and vitality and finally for immortality comes from. And then we should also make it concretely clear to ourselves that through our own behaviour we can add more life – and even much more life – at least to the existing years than has been considered normal up to now. But can we also add more years to our life? Can we not only influence the quality but also the quantity of our life by our behaviour?

Concerning this, let's have another look at the mentioned experiment with the rats that were fed the typical diet of various human cultures. It was conducted in the first half of the last century by the British scientific Sir Robert McCarrison, who spent many years in India and was surprised at the astonishing health and longevity of some ethnic groups, primarily the Hunza people, a small tribe then living in complete isolation in the Himalayas. Over the years the Hunza people were visited by several scientists, globetrotters and journalists so that we have some reports on their life. These reports concur about their great vitality, imposing appearance and outstanding health. No degenerative diseases, such as are omnipresent with us, were to be found in them. It was normal for them to live to be 100. The usual lifespan even amounted to 110 or 120 years, with some people living to 130. Even in old age, they still enjoyed excellent health and at 100 were still in full possession of their eyesight and teeth. Women of 80 were alleged to look like 40-year-old Americans and men of 90 or 100 still fathered children. Overweight was unknown and it was normal for them to work in the fields daily until the end of their days.

How is something like that possible? Or better expressed: How was something like that possible? For today the "accomplishments" of civilisation even seem to have caught up with this reclusive tribe. More recent travel reports write about alarming degenerative phenomena and developments, such as have already become "normal" with us. It was this very question that McCarrison wanted to get to the bottom of in his rat experiments. When he did an autopsy of the rats with a Hunza diet corresponding in age to a 50-year-old human he found nothing – no signs of heart disease, cancer, diabetes, stroke, osteoporosis, obesity, diseases of the bowel, kidneys or liver – nothing, absolutely nothing. You can imagine how much that surprised him, particularly in comparison with the other groups of rats, in which symptoms of disease and degenerative phenomena had occurred in abundance. Therefore he began a second experiment, in which he fed a group of rats the Hunza diet, continued this with their offspring and only took a few rats as random samples now and again to do an autopsy. In this way, he observed the proceedings over several generations and could not find any signs of degeneration, even in the long term.

Thus, their diet seems to have been a main factor in the Hunza people's exceptional health and longevity: it consisted mainly of fresh ingredients, contained almost no meat and was not too copious either. It is even reported that they often had to fast a few weeks in the spring when their store of food had run out before the new harvest was due. The second factor was their consciousness. For them it was quite normal to grow old in perfect health. If one of them had become ill at 80, they would have all been surprised and looked for the causes so as to eliminate them. On the other hand, if one of us becomes ill at 80, we regard it as normal. Nobody look for causes: on the contrary, everyone prepares themselves for the person concerned to maybe die soon. For "normally" people are already dead at that age.

The Hunza people certainly were not, nor are the prime example of perfect behaviour in harmony with the natural laws. They, too, made mistakes, which not least showed themselves in their rapid decline after contact with civilisation. But they still did many things better than we do today and therefore provide us with an example of what is possible. What conventional Ayurveda and also the Bible say, namely that the normal human lifespan is 120 years, may then be true. But doesn't the Bible also say that Adam lived to be 930 and fathered his son Seth at the age of 130, Seth lived to be 912, etc. up to Noah, who was said to have been 600 when the flood came? What are we to think of these indications of age? In the Ramayana from the Vedic tradition the indications of age even go into thousands of years! Whereas we are so proud that our life expectancy increases year by year and now has risen from 30 years in Roman times to around 80 years. What great credit to medical science! If it does not in fact bring us perfect health or at least real well-being, it at least lets us live longer and longer! Or maybe not? Let's imagine we are back in Roman times for a moment or in the Middle Ages, when life expectancy was only about 30 years. In ancient Greece it was even less than 20 years. Who actually raised the children when most parents passed away a few years after giving birth to them? People did not become grown up earlier than now at that time and they even reached sexual maturity later. Nobody knew their grandparents at that time, as a 60-, 70-, or 80-year-old must have been so exotic as a 110- or 130-year-old today. Nevertheless, old people appear in all literary works, as if they were the order of the day. There seems to be something wrong here.

We should better look into the matter, as it is not insignificant in determining our notion of normality today. How do we actually get the life expectancy, or more correctly, the average life expectancy? As the name already says, it is an average of the number of years people have lived when they die. As an example, for the sake of simplicity, let's take a small ethnic group, in which 13 people die in a particular year. One is 100 and the other 12 are only one month old. That is not even so absurd, for child and infant mortality used to be considerably higher than today. Now we add up all the ages and come to a total of 101 years. We now have to divide this number by the total number of dead people to get the average amount: $101 \div 13 = 7.77$: the average life expectancy in this ethnic group was, thus, 7.77 years in the year concerned, i.e. people died at a statistical age of 7.77 although the only adult who died was 100 years old. The calculation is absolutely correct and exactly consistent with the facts: only the interpretation of the number needs to be quite different from the one we normally apply to life expectancy. It is, in fact, not the age at which people normally die but only a statistical average from all the dead people! And a high child mortality naturally lowers this average considerably, as we have ourselves just seen from our little example.

It was not any different in the past! The Greeks, the Romans and people in the Middle Ages lived to a normal age just like today – as long as they survived their first years of life. Most of them unfortunately died at or shortly after birth, thus pushing the arithmetic average down. But once the children were 4 or 5 years old, they were out of the danger zone and on average lived to be just as old us today. That can be proved without doubt by all old chronicles and literary documents. The increase in life expectancy therefore does not express that people are living to be older and older but that fewer and fewer – particularly children – die prematurely. And that is less to the credit of medical research than to better hygiene at delivery.

As far as general health is concerned, there is even rather an opposite trend to be registered. Whereas people in earlier centuries used to still be healthy as they got older and, in particular, kept their mental freshness, today people get seriously ill earlier and earlier. There are increasing incidences of cardiovascular problems, heart attacks and cancer as early as in the twenties and thirties and even children are more and more frequently affected. While it was still "normal" some years ago to get cancer at an advanced age and maybe die from it, the age barrier has now been broken and we even frequently hear of young people dying of cancer. This development has probably not yet affected the statistics because, at the same time, the technical procedures for artificially preserving life are being further and further perfected. But are weeks or months dependent on an artificial lung or an artificial kidney really what we understand by a longer life? Certainly not, and it is not for nothing that many young people signal their refusal when we speak of a long life. They would rather die earlier than languish away in such a manner and then be switched out of life in a degrading way.

In conclusion, let's consider another extremely memorable example from the England of the 17th century, when the average life expectancy was only 30 years. In 1635, King Charles I invited a farmer called Thomas Parr from the county of Shropshire to his court. There was evidence that Thomas Parr had been baptised in 1483 and was therefore 152 years old. Documents exist proving that he inherited the farm from his father in 1518 at the age of 35 and married in 1563 at the age of 80 and for the second time in 1605 at the age of 122. With his first wife he had a son and a daughter, who both died as children. Furthermore, there is a church record stating that he had to do public penance at the age of 105 because he had been unfaithful to his wife and fathered a child out of wedlock. His advice for a long life was: "Keep your head cool by temperance and your feet warm by exercise. Rise early, go soon to bed, and if you want to grow fat [prosperous] keep your eyes open and your mouth shut."

Charles I was very taken with Thomas's lively intelligence and excellent memory and invited him to live in his palace in London to the end of his days. Thomas accepted the offer, sold his farm, but dropped dead only a few weeks later during a court banquet. In his great surprise, Charles I ordered his court surgeon William Harvey to carry out an autopsy, which indicated the cause of death to be "an acute digestive disorder," provoked by "unaccustomed abuse of food." At the king's orders, Thomas was buried in Westminster Abbey. He was 152 years and 9 months old and had seen the reigns of 10 kings during his lifetime. This true story gives us a considerably more authentic insight into the life of the past centuries than the misinterpreted average life expectancies. Above all, it shows us in an exemplary way the difference between the simple population and the court nobility. Ordinary people, who did not have much and did not live in abundance, were thus healthy, vital and always lived to a good age with physical and mental freshness.

However, the nobility, who lived in affluence and tedium, were afflicted with all kinds of complaints already in their youth and went through considerable physical and mental degeneration until they died relatively young. The ten kings Thomas survived show this clearly.

The fatal thing was and is, however, that normality was not determined by the population as a whole but by the nobility, and ordinary people had always wanted to be able to live like the nobility. Thomas had to pay for this error with his life after a short time and today our eyes should also be opened to this inverted reality. It is high time to recognise where our friend is and where our foe.

In summary, we can say that our body and nature provide all the conditions for making the dream of a long life in health and wisdom come true. We just have to change our attitude and our behaviour fundamentally.

Even various scientists say that physiologically it ought to be possible to live to 130 or even 150. They thereby take the present functioning state of our physiology as a basis without considering our consciousness and possible, so far undiscovered development potential. But if we take into account the possibility that mechanisms are concealed in ourselves that can not only effect a gradual improvement of our current state but an absolute quantum leap, the written records from old traditions move into the sphere of the conceivable, though not into the sphere of the imaginable.

To make what is conceivable tangible, many far-reaching developments in body and mind are necessary, all of which, however, begin with the same first step. If we take this first step and then continue with the second and third, etc. at the proper time, we get on a path that is sure to lead us to better health, increased mental clarity and a longer and more fulfilling life. Where it will continue to, how many years we will live and what facilities in us will be revived greatly depend on our consistency, our will and our conviction. Limits are only set by ourselves through our behaviour and consciousness.

For by nature everything – including eternity - is in our hands. In our real existence as the crown of creation in God's image, we are not subject to any restrictions through our body and can consciously discard it ourselves in full possession of our physical vitality and mental clarity at the due point in time in harmony with our destiny. Besides that, we have unrestricted access to true eternity beyond our physical shell. But in order to experience and realise all this, a profound change in our consciousness and behaviour is indispensable.

4. Being conscious

At the end of a presentation on meditation in a small town in the Swabian Alb a young woman came to the Darshana. She was called Martha, at the end of her twenties, of medium height, had a good figure and a pretty face but made a sad impression. She said she did not feel good and lacked joy in life. Although she actually had everything and had no recognisable reason to be dejected, she was depressed. Her doctor spoke of endogenous depression and had already referred her to a psychiatrist. However, before consulting the psychiatrist, she wanted to hear what AyurVeda Ritam recommended in this case. I congratulated her on this step, for classical doctors are helpless concerning the phenomenon of endogenous depression and – as with so many problems of body and mind –the only thing that occurs to them is to try administering some medication, in this case psychotropic drugs, which in general, however, are very likely mess up the nervous system completely. Having a name for a disease is, in fact, far from understanding it or being able to provide any help in healing it.

But AyurVeda Ritam understands this problem very well. I explained that it is an expression of the soul, which does not feel well in the body because the latter does not provide it with the functional foundation it actually needs or because it cannot pursue its purpose in the body. Since the soul has the world of emotions as its functional mechanism, it expresses this malaise via the emotions, hoping that the mind will recognise that something is not in order and go in search of a solution. Thus, the actual problem is the mind, which has gone in the wrong direction or is so foggy that it does not pay any heed to the soul's emotional expressions or overrides it with intellectual arguments. In this way, it holds on to modes of behaviour which are bad for us because it has a different conviction intellectually. We, thus, have to help our mind let go and become open and free again so as to be able to reorient its attitude and behaviour and bring it into harmony with the needs of body and soul. Ritam Samation is the perfect aid for this, as I had already explained in my presentation the previous day, for it first of all releases the mind from its conscious level of thinking, in which it is imprisoned day in and day out, leading to the elimination of old, unresolved impressions which disrupt its normal, unencumbered functioning and finally giving impulses for a reorientation and restructuring of our patterns of thinking and consciousness. Hence, my recommendation to Martha was to make sure to attend the Ritam Samation course scheduled to take place two weeks later.

But, besides that, I recommended her another thing. For endogenous depressions often have an absolutely concrete, directly tangible cause – meat consumption. When an animal is taken to be slaughtered, it feels exactly what is coming to it. Therefore in the minutes before its death it releases an enormous quantity of stress and fear hormones, which circulate throughout its body. A person who eats this body also eats these hormones, which naturally continue their impact of stress and fear in the person's body – without any recognisable external reason. Therefore my second recommendation is to eliminate meat, fish, eggs, mushrooms and algae from the diet, preferably immediately.

The Ritam Samation course took place two weeks later. Martha appeared punctually to be instructed and entered the room with a smile on her face. Without being asked, she immediately told me how well she felt. For some days she had had an awareness of life that she had not had for a long time. Straight after the Darshana she had put my recommendation into practice and categorically removed meat, fish, eggs, mushrooms from her diet.

"At first I really had to think a lot and look for what I should and can eat," she reported, "but once I realised what an enticing variety of other foods there is, I am greatly enjoying trying and getting to know them and don't know if I'll ever be able to eat everything nature provides."

But the crucial thing had been that she had already felt much lighter after just a few days. As if a stone had been sliding off her soul, her mental state had improved from day to day and she had actually experienced happiness and joy many times.

"I have to confess," she told me with an arch look, "that for a few days I even thought I needn't attend the course now because my depression was as good as gone. But then I thought: 'If that little piece of advice to stop eating meat already had such an impact, whatever will the meditation do to help me!' And so I'm actually even more encouraged to take part. For now I know from personal experience that you aren't promising too much!"

I couldn't help smiling. The refreshing way she said it did not in any way let it be suspected what state I had got to know her in just a few days before.

Yes, it was a small piece of advice with a great impact! Or conversely, a small mistake with a devastating impact. That is why most people do not attach any great importance to meat consumption, as if to say: "A little meat or sausage can't really be so bad!" or "If you don't overdo it and eat large amounts, there is surely no objection to it"! But we must not forget that we eat this "little amount" three times a day, 7 days a week, 52 weeks a year and have been doing that for 30, 40, 50 or 60 years! In this way the smallest amount of poison leads to fatal poisoning.

"But meat isn't poison! That comparison simply goes too far!" Now I can literally hear the objections raised at this point in every one of my presentations. "You don't have to be a fanatic! Everything in moderation! I can just about understand that you attach such great importance to diet, but why is it necessary to demonise meat to that extent?!" When I hear such words I always have to think of a presentation that Samuk Deda, the founder of AyurVeda Ritam, gave in a small Bavarian town some years ago. When it was a question of food, he spoke of "carcass eaters", thereby provoking a real uproar in the audience. People gave vent to their displeasure at this "demonisation of meat" using coarse expressions and furious gestures. "Meat gives strength!", "We don't want to look like weak grain eaters!" and similar shouts echoed through the room. Some of the keenest ranters had stood up and challenged Samuk Deda directly.

Any other presenter would probably have fled in this situation, but Samuk stood unmoved. It was clear to him that he could only master the situation by taking the offensive. So he calmly took off his jacket and made a gesture to the audience, indicating they should now pay attention. For it was no longer possible to make himself understood with words because of the loud background noise. Then he did a handstand, remained in the position for some minutes and even walked a few steps on his hands. The audience became silent. Nobody had expected that. Samuk used the silence to invite his listeners to do the same. When nobody reacted, he asked for a volunteer to compete with him in arm wrestling. After a short silence, a burly, bearded young man did, in fact, raise his hand. Samuk asked him to come to the front and when they shook hands Samuk, who was a head shorter and distinctly slighter, looked downright lost beside him. He asked what the man's name was, then they sat down at a table opposite each other and clasped hands with their elbows on the table. There was breathless suspense in the room. In contrast to a few minutes before, you could have now heard a pin drop. Then they began. Both of them pressed for all they were worth, but their arms did not move even a millimetre. But, after a few moments, the man from the audience started to give way slightly, then more and more, and a short time later Samuk had pressed his arm down on to the table. A murmur went round the room. The two men repeated the whole thing with the other arm and the result was the same. Then Samuk addressed the audience:

"Now we don't want to make a real competition out of this little challenge. The conditions for that aren't optimal either. But I would like to thank Hans. He pressed excellently and I would be happy to do a return match later. What I actually wanted to demonstrate to you is that meat has nothing to do with strength or even stamina. How old are you, Hans?" "25" was the answer. "You see," Samuk went on, "I'm 60."

He thus had the situation under control again. The audience now listened to him with even greater openness than before and so he was able to explain in detail that although the expression "carcass eaters" may not be normal, it is still correct. "Carcass" in fact means nothing but a "dead animal's body" and that is exactly what people everywhere are consuming. Strictly speaking, we should even use the expression "carrion eaters" for the meat is not fresh when it gets to the table but is at least days and mostly weeks old and even much older in sausages and ham.

What are those mechanisms which provoke disgust and revulsion in most people when they hear the words "carcass" or "carrion"? And why do these mechanisms only work with those words and not when parts of the dead animal's body are actually lying on a plate and being pushed into someone's mouth? It is not a question of demonising anything but simply of calling a spade a spade, giving information about what meat means for the body and what fish, eggs, mushrooms and algae have to do with it. Everyone has to draw conclusions about this for themselves, for we all have our free will. Nobody ought to be forced into anything, but you can certainly only decide freely when you have the necessary information. That has something to do with consciousness. For only when we know what we are doing and what the consequences of our doings are can we act consciously and be conscious. Before that, we follow whatever patterns of behaviour out of ignorance, thoughtlessness or sheer habit, without being at all clear about their consequences.

So let us analyse the issue of meat unemotionally and completely without reservations and together gain an insight into what goes on in our body. But for this we will begin at just the other end, namely with the minute creatures – bacteria and fungi – which are everywhere in our surroundings, in the air, in water and also in food. These microscopic beings are so ubiquitous that it is almost impossible to escape them. Every usable substance is immediately and directly attacked by them so that the traces of their metabolic and reproductive activities are soon manifest. With organic substances this is either mildew visible to the naked eye or fermentation and putridness. In wounds or body openings, in contrast, they are noticeable as infections. It was not until the 19th century that modern man realised that such phenomena do not come from food or the body opening itself but from outside and can therefore also be prevented by disinfectant measures. That was the birth of hygiene, one of the greatest breakthroughs in the improvement of general health, fighting infectious diseases and the increase in life expectancy. We have already spoken about this in connection with child mortality.

Our body handles these creatures very pragmatically. It lets the useful ones live, even allowing them to enter the body and providing them with ideal living conditions. In contrast, it holds the ones that harm it in check by means of its immune system. For this purpose, all the surfaces of the body connected with the outside world are coated with a fine energetic defensive film, the so-called ojas. We usually do not notice this ojas unless it collapses or is irritated somewhere. For the affected areas are then attacked by fungi, bacteria or viruses or react abnormally to other substances: in this case we speak of allergies as is well known. The fact that such problems occur more and more frequently can be ascribed to our behaviour itself. For no defensive system can withstand the innumerable toxins in our clothing, detergents and toiletries in the long term.

So-called thrush, an oral and anal mycosis mostly appearing in both places, is frequently to be found in small children. Many people have similar experiences with herpes, a virus infection in the oral and genital regions. We can recognise from this that these regions of the body at diametrically opposed locations are in fact connected with each other, namely through the digestive tract.

The crucial thing is that the body cannot manage to keep off the harmful microscopic organisms or viruses either. For they are really ubiquitous. The body can only keep them in check, which, however requires constant control. But if even only a minor weakness occurs, the troublemakers can immediately get a foothold and spread. Many people have had this experience with the herpes virus, where a slight weakening of the ojas in the oral cavity due to too much sun, aggressive foods or chemical substances is sufficient and "the herpes is there". In reality it was there the entire time but was just kept in check by our ojas. Women often have the same experience with mycosis in the vagina. There a trifle suffices, often such a minor thing that the woman does not recognise the cause, and the natural vaginal flora is disrupted so that fungi can settle there.

However, this example helps us to understand another important principle. The most effective and, at the same time, gentlest remedy with such a vaginal mycosis does not, in fact, consist in fighting the fungus but in reinforcing the natural vaginal flora by supplying lactobacilli. This can be done in the form of suppositories but also quite simply by inserting some fresh natural yoghurt into the vagina. At the same time, it should be ensured that optimal living conditions are no longer offered for the fungus. Fungi need moisture and trapped heat, which they get plenty of under panties and tights made of synthetic material. On the other hand, they are sensitive to fresh air and sunshine. That is why these are the best "fire-fighting methods" for fungi of all kinds, whether on the feet, in the genital region or somewhere else on the skin. In general, this principle regulates the spread of the miniscule creatures. For the fact that all types – lactobacilli, putrefactive bacteria, yeast, mould – are constantly omnipresent means that every single organic substance is attacked by all of them simultaneously. The ones that find the best living conditions – related to the combination of nutrients, air, light, temperature, milieu, etc. – then reproduce the fastest and dominate. All the others perish and are suppressed. Humans have been making use of this for centuries when preserving food in lactic acid, particularly in making sauerkraut. There, the desired cultures are lactobacilli, which is why in the first stage all the other bacteria have to be suppressed by adding sufficient salt, strictly excluding air, correct temperature, etc. Once the lactobacilli have gained a foothold, there is no chance for the other bacteria anymore. But if something goes wrong in the first stage, the sauerkraut is irretrievably lost.

With this understanding, we will now consider various foods and other organic substances. First of all, it is clear that a fungal attack – whether from mould or yeast – can only take place when there is a moist milieu with little air circulating. So if we ensure conditions with fresh air and light, the fungi are at a disadvantage from the start. Under conditions with sufficient warmth and moisture the lactobacilli will win with most foodstuffs – provided no immune mechanisms are active. Hence, intact fruits will not be attacked at all as their peel guarantees protection until its intactness is destroyed by damage, cutting or suchlike. Concerning this, it is also to be noted that the actual lactic acid fermentation only takes place when air is excluded. In contrast, the process is somewhat different in the presence of oxygen, and no lactic acid is formed. Therefore different processes take place on the surface from inside the food.

Observation shows us that there are only five categories of foods which are not attacked by lactobacilli but by putrefactive bacteria. Those are meat, fish, eggs, mushrooms and algae. If we let these stand open for a few days, they start to stink and rot and anyone who then eats them suffers acute food poisoning. This is all the result of the metabolism of the putrefactive bacteria, which are responsible for decay everywhere in nature and produce ptomaine (cadaveric poisons).

As we saw previously, the bacterial attack occurs immediately and directly after the destruction of natural immune protection. So as soon as a fruit is damaged, part of a plant torn off, an animal killed, an egg opened, a mushroom or an alga picked, all kinds of bacteria and spores settle on it, with the ones finding the best conditions and nourishment quickly gaining the upper hand. Those are lactobacilli in the case of almost all foodstuffs and, on the other hand, putrefactive bacteria in the case of meat, fish, eggs, mushrooms and algae. If we eat such foods, the cultures established on them find ideal living conditions in our intestines – warmth, moisture and nourishment. In this respect, the type of bacteria or fungi is not significant. For the major part of them pass through our stomach largely undamaged. Neither does it make any difference how long they have been sitting on our food. For at the moment we consume the food at the latest we destroy their integrity and enable micro-organisms to settle on them. In this way, bacteria gradually settle in each person's gut after their birth so that we normally have 10 times as many bacteria in our gut as cells in our body. A healthy gut flora is composed of some 400 different species of bacteria, of which lactobacilli are one of the most important. But, in principle, all types of micro-organisms are to be found, as they come into the gut again and again with food, and the same principle as mentioned above applies. i.e. those which find the best conditions more easily establish themselves. Our diet, thus, has a huge influence on our gut flora, since it, firstly, provides food for specific types of bacteria but not for others and, secondly, it may also contain toxins in the form of antibiotics, preservatives and other food additives, which severely decimate some species of bacteria.

What is the task of the gut flora in our body? For the bacteria in the gut do not get food and ideal living conditions from us for nothing. They also render us services in return. We call such a situation symbio- sis or mutual dependence for the benefit of both sides. The gut bacte- ria are an essential part of our metabolic system. For they metabolise some things that our stomach and intestines have not digested or are not able to digest at all. For example, the actually indigestible ballast and fibre constitute an important source of nutrition for the gut flora, which make valuable vitamins from them as products of their metab- olism. In particular, the important group of B vitamins is produced by the gut bacteria in a healthy gut.

However, problems occur when the gut flora is disrupted. For then bacteria or even fungi that generate products of metabolism harmful to our body gain the upper hand, constantly releasing toxins. These toxins have their initial impact on the gut's immune system and the in- testinal mucosa. Approximately 10% of the cells in the gut are namely lymphatic immune cells, which ensure that foreign bodies and pests are eliminated. If they are weakened or destroyed by the toxins creat- ed, the result is a considerable impairment of our immune protection. The next thing the toxins do is to weaken the natural control and fil- tering function of the gut wall itself, which admits more and more sub- stances which should actually be kept back as they are harmful to our organism. Finally, the toxins even penetrate the gut wall and via the blood and lymph system get into the entire body, where they lead to deposits, inflammatory processes or allergic immune reactions. The fatal thing is that the entire process takes place in a creeping manner. In general, the quantities of toxins put into circulation are not so large that we immediately become acutely ill and notice that something is wrong. Instead, the small quantities remain unnoticed for a long time but, nevertheless, have consequences which spread more and more and become worse until suddenly disruptions occur somewhere, which we mostly do not connect with their actual cause. Usually we simply consider them to be inevitable accompaniments of the aging process or normal wear and tear due to long-term strain. Since such explanations stop us from going in search of the causes, we naturally do not correct anything in our mistakes and the process continues up to the bitter end.

Let's follow what happens to a meal of meat in our digestive system. First of all, it is to be noted that, unlike fruit and vegetables, meat does not contain any digestive enzymes, so that our stomach has to produce strong hydrochloric acid to break it down, which it manages more or less well, depending on how the meat has been cooked, how thoroughly it has been chewed and what other food has been eaten together with it. As meat, unlike most plant foods, is very dry, the acid is diluted again in the stomach by the necessary liquid drunk in addition to the food so that the meat is mostly not completely broken down. In the subsequent digestive process the acid has to be neutralised again, taking calcium from the body.

In the gut the meat then provides food for the putrefactive bacteria, which develop their activity and produce ptomaine. Although the gut attempts to protect itself from these toxins by increasing its production of protective mucous, the gut flora and also the gut wall suffer damage. A higher percentage particularly of the acid products of metabolism from the meat protein, the very long saturated fatty acid molecules, cholesterol and also the ptomaine penetrate the gut wall, placing a great burden on the liver, which tries to continue processing and breaking all that down. This generates uric acid, and partly urea as well, which, in turn, place a great strain on the kidneys and rob the body of considerable amounts of minerals during the elimination of these products.

However, as a pound of meat produces more than twice as much uric acid as our system can eliminate on one day, a large part of it remains in the body and, on account of its very low degree of water solubility, forms crystals in various places: these damage the surrounding tissue similarly to sharp needles, causing pain. The consequences are kidney stones, rheumatism and gout. Furthermore, the long saturated fatty acid molecules and the foreign cholesterol thicken the blood, leading to higher blood pressure and reduced blood flow. Besides, they tend to stick together and deposit themselves primarily on the inner walls of the blood vessels, where these have been damaged by the acids generated. This leads to a narrowing and hardening of the blood vessels. In the long term, all this results in gall stones, arteriosclerosis, heart attacks, strokes and, overall, in an impaired supply of nutrients to many parts of the body.

Meanwhile, the piece of meat moves on through the gut, with its progress being very slow because of the complete lack of fibre. Moreover, some undigested remains always get stuck to the villi together with the hardening protective mucous, so that an increasingly thick, impenetrable, sticky layer of excrement is formed in the course of time, making it harder and harder for the nutrients to get into the body. Autopsies have shown that it has now become normal to have 4 or 5 kg of old excremental remains sticking to the villi in your gut. These naturally provide an ideal breeding ground for parasites and make it harder for the food to pass through the gut, which, in turn, leads to chronic constipation. Overall, regular consumption of meat, fish, eggs, mushrooms and algae creates a stable nutritional base for putrefactive bacteria in the gut, therefore increasingly suppressing the natural gut flora so that their task of producing vitamins can no longer be fulfilled.

When the meat remains finally end their journey through the gut after long hours of effort, their excretion is always linked to the now characteristic stench produced by the putrefactive bacteria. Moreover, the body also eliminates part of the toxins ingested through the skin in the course of time, additionally resulting in the typical vapour exuding from meat eaters.

If we consider plant-based food, on the other hand, it is characterised by being much more digestible and partly even containing enzymes conducive to digestion. This means that much less effort is required of the stomach, pancreas and liver to digest this food. In the gut it is primarily metabolised by a healthy gut flora, which does not generate any harmful substances and – in a healthy gut – even produces valuable vitamins. The products of metabolism are mainly alkaline here so that the body is not burdened with acidity and no calcium is needed to neutralise this. Moreover, this food functions as a broom due to its natural ballast material and cleans the gut walls instead of burdening them with deposits. In this way, rapid and easy excretion takes place at the same time.

If we realise all this, there is actually no reason to demonise meat. For it demonises itself, at least as food for humans. For anyone whose health is important to them and wants to get to know true health – which is what we are in quest of – has to categorically avoid meat, fish, eggs, mushrooms and algae. It is not enough only to reduce them, as then the putrefactive bacteria in our gut get food again and again. And since they do not starve if they get no food but only restrict their metabolism and reproduction, they can wait patiently for the next meal that provides them with food. Therefore the only possibility to keep them permanently in check is to give them absolutely nothing more to eat. Then the normal gut flora can slowly but surely regenerate itself and resume its metabolic activity. But at least 1½ years pass before this balance has been restored, with the time being lengthened by every new consumption of meat, fish, eggs, mushrooms or algae. Unfortunately it is so that every mouthful of meat, every egg and every mushroom provides food for the putrefactive bacteria, stimulating them to reproduce again and weakening the healthy gut flora.

Yet, conversely, it does not take 1½ years before you experience the impact of a change of diet. The first signs can appear very soon, as we have seen with Martha, whose psyche breathed a sigh of relief after just a few days. In her case, it was probably not only the fear and stress hormones from meat, but the toxic load in general which had caused her problems previously, and, above all, the thickened blood, which could not flow into the finest arteries at all any longer. This means that many regions of the body and particularly of the brain are not adequately supplied with nutrients and energy, which may lead to an actual emotional feeling of oppression and states of anxiety. Elli, whom I had recommended to stop eating meat, fish, eggs, mushrooms and algae besides cultivating hunger and Ritam Samation, also had her initial experience very soon, as we have already seen.

However, some people seem to have a contrary experience at the beginning. They report that something is lacking, they feel hungry or do not have as much energy as before and are therefore inclined to break off the experiment immediately. Such experience is, however, mostly due to errors in the change of diet, which we will discuss in a moment. Therefore, everyone should give themselves at least six months in total before deciding about the success or failure of a change of diet. Only after this time can you judge your experience reliably and draw a balance. That is also completely without risk, for you can return to your old diet without further ado if your experience advises this. Likewise, nobody will suffer a deficiency during that time but rather enrichment from a new experience.

But what is actually the situation with the deficiencies that people – and doctors as well – so insistently warn about? And shouldn't there be some other indications in nature that we are in reality vegetarians if meat is actually so bad for humans? Let's simply have a look at typical carnivores and typical herbivores in the animal kingdom and see which category we humans are rather to be assigned to. However, with herbivores we have to, strictly speaking, distinguish between frugivores and grazers.

First of all, from an external point of view, it strikes us at once that carnivores are equipped with full facilities for procuring their food – claws, talons and carnassial teeth. They move horizontally for speed and can see well at night. It is different with herbivores. They have no claws or carnassial teeth and cannot see anything in the dark. In contrast, frugivores walk upright and have grasping hands so as to be able to pick and collect their food from trees.

The differences are also to be seen in their mouths: carnivores have pointed molars that do not meet when biting and are optimal for pulling meat apart, few salivary glands and acid saliva without the enzyme ptyalin for digesting starch.

Moreover, they can only move their jaws up and down. Frugivores, on the other hand, have flat molars for grinding food, a lot of salivary glands and alkaline saliva for predigesting starch. They can also move their jaws sideways and thus grind their food properly. Interestingly, typical omnivores, such as bears, have both types of molars – pointed and flat – at the same time.

As is to be expected, other distinct differences are to be found in the digestive systems: carnivores have a small round stomach with 10 times more hydrochloric acid in their gastric juices. Their intestines are short – only 3 – 5 times as long as their bodies – and smooth so that food does not stay long in them and their liver can produce much more uricase and thus cope with 10 – 15 times more uric acid. Besides that, they can themselves produce vitamin C, which is, among other things, important for absorbing iron. In contrast, frugivores have a long stomach with a complicated structure and only a little hydrochloric acid and pepsins for digesting protein in their gastric juice. Their intestines are 10 – 12 times as long as their body, very intertwined and endowed with a large surface, on account of the large number of villi in the intestinal wall, and their liver can only eliminate uric acid created by the body itself. They have to take in vitamin C regularly in their food.

With regard to excretion, it is striking that carnivores have acid urine and no pores or sweat glands in their skin. They regulate their temperature via their tongues. In contrast, frugivores have alkaline urine and millions of pores and sweat glands in their skin.

From these few properties, we can already see that typical carnivores do not have the above-mentioned problems with the consumption of meat. They can decompose meat protein and, on top of that, even sinews and bones completely, can cope with the uric acid produced, do not need fibre for digestion due to their smooth gut walls and can better manage the putrefaction process because of their shorter intestines, apart from the fact that the ptomaine is much less or not at all toxic for them. The acidic products of metabolism are normal for their organism, as can be seen from their urine, and saturated fatty acids and cholesterol are no problem for them either, as an investigation by the University of Iowa shows in addition. In it dogs were given half a pound of butter with their meat ration over a longer period, which was obviously not a problem for them, as they did not develop any signs of arteriosclerosis. In contrast, rabbits showed changes in their artery walls after a short time, when cholesterol was added to their food. Monkeys which were fed egg yolk also soon developed encrusted arteries.

However, in contrast to the typical carnivores in the animal kingdom, the human being has problems with all this and slowly but surely even perishes from it. This fact impressively underlines a human's unequivocal conformity with the physiological characteristics of typical frugivores. Moreover, as with all typical carnivores, the smell of blood and fresh meat should otherwise stimulate our appetites and the sight of a dead animal should make our mouths water. On the contrary, the reality is that nobody likes raw, unseasoned, uncooked or unfried meat but it provokes revulsion or even sometimes vomiting. Meat only becomes "palatable" when it gets in contact with fire and seasoning. So it is not the meat that we like the taste of but the extra ingredients and preparation. Yet, these can also be had with far fewer side-effects harmful to our health!

Is everyone now convinced that human beings are not carnivores, that meat is even harmful for them and should be completely eliminated from their diet?

Actually yes, but ...

Now we come to the arguments and motives which prevent even the most sensible – and often also the sickest – people from stopping eating meat. But basically it is not these arguments but a lack of conviction and a lack of will in their own consciousness. To justify this, the mind then seeks all kinds of alibis, in which it is, unfortunately, also strongly supported by today's medicine, science and the meat industry. For that reason, we should still treat the most important and frequent arguments or doubts and show that by no stretch of the imagination is there any way to bypass the truth.

First, there is the matter of the length of the gut. The human gut is, in fact, 6 – 7 m long, i.e. only 3 – 5 times as long as the body, which exactly corresponds to the relation to be found in typical carnivores. However, this calculation does not consider that with animals it is never the distance between head and feet but always between head and the lower end of the spine which is taken as a basis. If we take this as the basis for humans as well, we get a relation of 8 to 12, that of typical frugivores.

Nothing in this is changed by prehistoric people, who are commonly represented as hunters and therefore carnivores and, thus, have to serve as another popular alibi. But particularly with regard to human history, there are still so many fundamental question marks that everyone can bend their arguments to suit their purposes. Let's just imagine the old myths and written records were not figments of the imagination and our distant forebears led simple, devout lives with their physical and mental faculties functioning fully without the necessity of iron tools or monumental buildings for their posterity. What might we then still find today from such a very advanced civilization? Not the slightest trace! Thus, archaeological discoveries only give an extremely restricted picture of the past and it is still unclear whether the iron weapons and cave paintings actually have something to do with our origins or are already signs of early degeneration. At any rate, we could also propagate cannibalism as the healthy diet of primitive humans using the same arguments or refrain from all such threadbare arguments, preferring to orient ourselves towards mentally, spiritually and culturally outstanding personalities from the past, who were all vegetarians. Still today, our nearest relatives in the animal kingdom, the great apes, are, at any rate, impressive examples of strict frugivores brimming with strength and vitality.

The newly constructed theory of a diet specific to the blood group falls into the same category of alibis. It is, in fact, based on the genetic age of the various blood groups and on the picture archaeologists and anthropologists give us of our forebears. That is the reason why the oldest blood group "has to" belong to carnivores, for example. Any indication confirming the above-mentioned spiritually high civilisation instead of the primitive hunters would turn this entire dietary theory upside down and assign the same blood group to strict raw frugivores. So let's rather stay with concrete indications and experience than theories conjured arbitrarily out of a hat. And this experience shows unmistakably that people across all the blood groups get ill and die from uric acid, ptomaine and the other products of metabolism of meat. Meat, fish, eggs, mushrooms and algae are and remain no foods for humans, even in small amounts. When decades or generations of habits dispose someone to problems with a wholefood vegetarian diet, it is not a sign of genetic adaptation but of congenital biological degeneration on a large scale, which should be counteracted as rapidly as possible. Moreover, the reason for such alleged problems is mostly incorrect dealings with food and not an intolerance in principle. So it is really no wonder that fresh fruit starts to ferment in the digestive tract when it has to wait hours for the way to become free for its further digestion, as it is blocked by very hard to digest food rich in fat or protein. If large cultures of fermentation and yeast bacteria have additionally established themselves in the gut, due to a large consumption of sugar and white flour, they will also immediately metabolise the fruit into carbon dioxide and alcohol.

Thus, we again encounter the problem we addressed in chapter 2, that most people, in fact, concentrate exclusively on "what" and not "how" in eating. But someone who eats when they are not hungry inevitably wreaks havoc on their digestion, no matter whether they eat vegetarian food or meat, raw or cooked food, industrial or natural food. For when the stomach is still busy with the previous meal, how is it to manage to produce digestive juices in such a way that they suit both the new and the old food? This makes itself felt in a particularly drastic way with light and quickly digested foods, which actually go through the digestive system very fast. If they are held up because harder to digest foods from the previous or same meal have to be processed, they easily start to ferment, causing flatulence and bad odours. However, the fruit or vegetables are not to blame, but eating food in the wrong order or without being hungry. Therefore it has to be insistently emphasised once more – and everyone's experience will confirm it – that there are no problems with a wholefood vegetarian diet if you only eat when you are really hungry, chew adequately and stop eating when the food tastes best. This applies to every blood group and every type of constitution, for these are universal natural laws of our digestive system.

Of course, it is correct – and everyone must agree with this frequent objection – that vegetarian food alone does not mean a healthy diet. The word "vegetarian" is much too general and elastic. Moreover, again it only considers "what" and not "how." Therefore vegetarian food has to be redefined, namely in conformity with the principles of the human digestive system. Accordingly, – as we have just seen in detail –, all foods are vegetarian except meat, fish, eggs, mushrooms and algae, meaning, in other words, all those which are not attacked by putrefactive bacteria but by lactobacilli. Accordingly, the latter also include dairy products, for they become acidic and do not putrify. Nevertheless, we have to say a few more words about them later. The term "ovovegetarian" (i.e. vegetarians who also eat eggs) is, in contrast, a contradiction in terms, for eggs are to be virtually described as liquid meat. Also mushrooms, which are to be found in almost every popular vegetarian dish, do not belong here at all, as they trigger the same reaction as meat in the gut. This, on the other hand, also helps us understand why they are so popular in particular with people who have eliminated meat from their diet. But these people are unfortunately not aware that they are replacing one evil with another.

Next we must define what healthy food is, for that, in turn, is only a small part of the range of vegetarian foods. The only really healthy food is, in fact, pure, natural, unprocessed products which are consumed in keeping with physical needs. Accordingly, everything eaten without real hunger, in too large amounts or without adequate chewing is unhealthy in principle. Furthermore, it must be clear to us that any form of processing means denaturing, which devalues the food or provokes undesired side-effects in the body.

However, it is the case that our digestive system, our gut flora and our whole body require a certain time to adapt to a different diet. It probably takes our head, which is programmed by our year-long habits, the longest time. That is why nobody should try to climb the tenth rung of the ladder before the second one. That will always lead to bad relapses, frustration and possibly complete failure in the end. Let's rather climb the rungs one after the other and only go to the next when we have stabilised ourselves on the present one. If difficulties arise, we simply allow ourselves a bit more time, perhaps going back one rung but making a fresh attempt at the next opportunity. Only in this way will we become stable and progress most successfully.

In this process, our point of orientation should always be our body and its feedback, meaning, first and foremost, hunger as the unconditional requirement for any intake of food and reliable burner of any digestive problems. Furthermore, we pay attention to our body's signals and impulses, which dishes it feels attracted to and – and this is of the greatest importance! – what odours it generates after eating, on the toilet and in its perspiration. For any bad smell is a natural warning signal and any agreeable one an attractive enticement. When we cannot stand our own smell, it means that something in our body is not in order and we have to change something right away. The stench on the toilet, which has become customary everywhere, is a clear sign of unhealthy metabolic processes in the gut due either to the activity of putrefactive bacteria, unhealthy fermentation bacteria or yeast fungi. These, in turn, can only appear when we have given them food. And that is the point where we can and have to start. The food or food combination we have eaten in the meal concerned has been unmasked as wrong by our own body and we should not make this mistake again in future. It's as simple as that! And as we now know that meat, fish, eggs, mushrooms and algae constitute food for putrefactive bacteria and sugar and white flour the basis for fermentation, we can already eliminate the main problem factors from the start.

The often expressed concern about a one-sided diet is completely unfounded in this regard. For if you eat a wide selection of fruit, vegetables, herbs and grains from the garden of nature, you get everything the body needs in sufficient amounts and perfectly combined. Let's take time to consider the most frequently cited alleged issues of a vegetarian diet more exactly, namely an adequate supply of protein, calcium, iron and vitamin B 12. However, here we want to rely more on our common sense and the elementary rule of three than on official recommendations, which are rather marked by the scientific mind-set, lobbying by the industries concerned or the sickness of our society being considered normal. For example, in the last 50 years the official recommendation for daily protein consumption has been reduced to a fifth (!), the reason for which certainly does not lie in our body's functioning mode having changed but in the in those responsible gradually dawning out of deeper regions of ignorance.

For assessing the generally needed amounts of protein and also calcium mother's milk certainly provides a good guideline given by nature. For it is the natural food for a baby, which doubles its body weight within six months and needs a higher concentration of protein in its food for the necessary growth work than in its entire subsequent life.

The usual tables of ingredients are, however, unfortunately of very little use for comparing the values of various foods with each other. For they always give the ingredients in relation to the weight of the food concerned, that is in g or mg per 100 g or per kg of the food. But nobody gears their eating behaviour to the weight of a meal but rather to their hunger and feeling of satiation, which, in turn, corresponds to the energy content of the meal. In other words, everyone eats on average on one day the amount that contains as much energy as they use on that day. And the food tables are also generally interpreted so as to indicate how much of substance x a person would take up with their food if they only ate food y. In this case, they would cover their energy needs exclusively from food y and therefore eat as much of it until their hunger was stilled. That is why we need the ingredients in relation to the amount of energy in the food, i.e. in g or mg per kcal and not in relation to its weight. The usual misleading data are also the reason that in conventional tables foods containing water are sometimes at a great disadvantage over dry ones. For the amount of water drunk later to quench one's thirst should actually be added to the latter's weight, whereas it is contained in the former from the start.

If we convert the available data accordingly, we obtain surprising results. As a benchmark mother's milk contains 15 mg of protein per kcal, which is approximately the same amount as in papayas, plums or mandarins. Water melons contain 1.3 as much protein per kcal, carrots 1.6 as much, tomatoes 2.7 as much and pumpkins 3.3 as much.

It should be noted that our benchmark was the protein concentration for a baby, which has to build a huge amount of cells within a short time, whereas we adults only need protein for maintaining and renewing our body. In absolute terms, we naturally need more protein for our larger body, which is, after all, to the order of 100 times heavier. But we also use more energy so that the percentage of our protein requirements is lower.

So even a baby could cover its protein requirements from fruit without any problem. The percentage of protein in other fruit is also a little above or below that of mother's milk. We experience other surprises if we examine the upper part of the scale. Eggs contain 68 mg of protein per kcal, Edam cheese 70, white beans 71, beef 83 – just as much as iceberg lettuce! – soy beans 88, lettuce 91, broccoli 107, salmon 111, mushrooms 116, spinach 130, alfalfa sprouts 137, pork and chicken 150 each and spirulina algae 228. We can easily see from these figures – above all, from the examples of iceberg lettuce, broccoli, spinach and alfalfa sprouts –, that the prejudice regarding the much higher protein content of meat, fish, eggs, mushrooms and algae is only correct to a limited extent. Although they top the table and considerably contribute to the general oversupply of protein because of their large share in the average diet, we can obtain similarly high amounts of protein without difficulty from a purely vegetarian diet. Thus, the protein requirements of an average adult with slight physical movement would be covered if they only ate either honeydew melons, apricots or potatoes, and those of an average athlete and even of a bodybuilder weighing 75 kg, who spends three hours daily on training with exercise equipment, if they only ate either celery, pumpkins, cucumbers or cabbage. It even shows that you would have to make a downright effort to fall short of the recommended amounts of protein. For example, 3000 kcal of pumpernickel bread or noodles without egg already contain over 100 g of protein. A person who consumes sufficient calories therefore automatically takes in enough protein as well.

All that would certainly be a very one-sided diet and it is not intended to show a realistic way of eating here either. It should only make clear that the so often cited lack of protein in vegetables and fruit is nothing more than a myth. It is the same with the so-called biological value of protein, which is supposed to express how many of the essential amino-acids which the body cannot synthesise itself are contained in a specific food. Meat, fish and, above all, eggs also rank first here, but this data has no great practical value for the everyday diet as nobody can systematically eat only one or very few foods one-sidedly over a long period. But if you eat various foods with a lower value, the essential amino-acids contained in them complement each other and allow the body to make its own proteins without any problem. Contrary to some recommendations, it is not necessary at all to take in all essential amino-acids in one meal or even on the same day, for the body is intelligent enough and stores them to be accessed according to need.

We often hear meat-eaters say that all the combining and varying of foods is too complicated for them and that they therefore prefer to be on the safe side by regularly eating the very protein-rich meat. However, this argument in quite clearly based on a lack of reflection (or on the desperate search for an alibi). For a varied diet is a completely natural thing, which is automatically everybody's goal without any effort alone for reasons of taste. Due to its one-sidedness, meat, in particular, requires varied supplements. Nobody would be able to stand even one week eating meat exclusively – without a piece of bread, a potato or a vegetable to better get the meat down and digest it. In contrast, you can live from exclusively fruit and vegetables without any problem your whole life long – as many people do – without deficiencies, without constant reflection or complicated combining.

Contrary to widespread concern and innumerable warnings, it has unfortunately been shown that today's customary diet does not engender a lack but a considerable excess of protein. Thus, an average person eats 2 – 3 times the official recommendation for protein – and this official amount is already much too high. But unfortunately too much protein is not simply an excess that the body easily disposes of. It, in fact, presents a real problem and is the cause of numerous degenerative diseases. On the one hand, excessive protein, in principle, accelerates growth and development of humans and animals, which we can, in fact, actually observe: people in the Western industrialised countries are becoming taller and taller and the age at which girls mature sexually has decreased from 17 to 12 in the hundred years from 1875 to 1975. At the same time, this development extends to the whole of life, thus also considerably shortening lifespan. The eskimos and the Russian Kurgi tribes have the largest proportion of meat in their diet and the shortest lifespan of sometimes only 30 years. In contrast, we have already got to know the Hunza tribe, who lived almost completely as vegetarians and had a longevity almost inconceivable to us. But the main problem is the metabolism of protein itself, as an excess of protein is not used as structural building material but as a supplier of energy. The digestion of protein, however, represents a considerable burden on the liver and kidneys, leading to their enlargement and diseases such as diabetes, hypoglycaemia, hepatitis, kidney problems and, in general, to acidosis of the blood. The resulting acidic products of metabolism can only be neutralised and excreted using a large amount of minerals, with the body losing huge amounts of calcium. It is, thus, not chance that there is an increased incidence of osteoporosis in those countries where an excess of protein is consumed. Paradoxically, calcium is the very argument repeatedly used against a strictly vegetarian diet, above all when it also excludes dairy products.

So we will have a look at calcium, again taking as the benchmark mother's milk, which provides the baby with sufficient calcium for the growth of its bones and development of its teeth. It contains 0.46 mg of calcium per kcal. That is approximately equivalent to strawberries, fresh figs or kiwis. Papayas and carrots contain 1.3 times as much, oranges and pumpkins 1.8 times as much, cucumbers and radishes 2.3 times as much. Spirulina algae contain approximately the same amount of calcium per kcal as mother's milk, whereas eggs only contain 60%, mushrooms 45% and meat even only between 6 and 15%. Top of the list are sesame and broccoli with 1.7 mg per kcal, milk with 1.9 mg – just as much as in cabbage (!) -, cheese with 2 mg, celery with 2.5 mg, lettuce with 3.8 mg, rhubarb with 4.1 and spinach with 2.5 mg, almost ten times the content of mother's milk. In this case as well, the myth of the necessity of dairy products and meat cannot be maintained. On the contrary, the highly concentrated and hard to digest protein in dairy products takes more calcium from the body for its digestion than it provides at the same time.

Finally, we want to take a look at the amounts of iron, which also frequently serve as arguments for meat in our diet. If we also convert the food tables to the energy content here, we get astonishing results. Mother's milk in fact contains no more than 0.43 µg (microgram = 0.00043 mg) per kcal, cow's milk only 0.78 µg. Every type of fruit contains at least five times as much and some fruits and seeds even much more. For example, strawberries contain 30 times as much iron as mother's milk does, red peppers 40 times as much, cucumbers 47 times as much, pumpkins 70 times as much, courgettes and green beans 86 times as much, mulberries 100 times as much and green peas 115 as much. Top-scorers are potatoes with 55.9 µg per kcal, lettuce with 77.8 µg, spirulina algae with 107 µg, spinach with 123 µg and parsley with 172 µg. Beef has 8.4 µg – that is about two-thirds the amount in strawberries –, pork and chicken even only 5.5 µg, roughly as much as water melons. With 3.9 µg, salmon contains as much iron as grapes, with their 7.8 µg, eggs contain somewhat more than hazelnuts. Mushrooms still score better with 42 µg iron per kcal, but they do not even quite match mulberries. In addition to all this is the fact that the body needs vitamin C to be able to absorb the iron from food properly, and the actually so highly praised suppliers of iron from the animal world contain almost none.

Thus, we again come to the point that the foods the body absorbs do not primarily depend on their quantity in the diet but on the functioning of the digestive system. This, in turn, is obstructed in its ability to absorb iron by red wine, black tea, coffee and cocoa (in chocolate as well), in addition to the already mentioned negative accompaniments of our wrong diet. It should therefore give food for thought that the USA of all countries, which ranks first in the per capita consumption of meat, also leads in the number of cases of anaemia. For the same reason, the officially recommended amounts of iron in our diet should be submitted to a serious examination. An alarming correlation between excessive amounts of iron in the blood and heart attacks has already been established. Moreover, Alzheimer sufferers have been found to have an abnormally high amount of iron in their brain.

At the end of our considerations, we now come to the much cited vitamin B12, the largest and most complex of all vitamin molecules. It is synthesised exclusively by micro-organisms, in uncontaminated soil, in the fermentation of vegetables and in the digestive systems of animals and humans. Therefore it is to be found in the roots of organic vegetable, in sauerkraut, tofu, soy sauce or similar fermented foods and in meat. The actual supplying with this vitamin, however, takes place naturally in the activity of the gut flora in a healthy gut. There the gut bacteria, which we have already spoken about, particularly in the large intestines, produce this vital vitamin for our body in an adequate amount. A person who eats a healthy vegetarian diet therefore does not need to worry about vitamin B12, as they cultivate their gut flora in the best way through their diet. But someone who eats meat, fish, eggs, mushrooms or algae feeds the putrefactive bacteria in their gut, which spread at the expense of the normal, healthy gut flora, disrupting the latter's functioning and sometimes even bringing it to a halt.

Here, we recognise a tragic paradox in the entire diet discussion. Through their diet people themselves generate the very thing most of them fear and the reason they do not want to switch to a vegetarian diet– malnutrition and undersupply with just those substances for which meat and dairy products are allegedly necessary. In particular, meat, fish, eggs, mushrooms and algae cultivate the putrefactive bacteria in the gut which destroy natural synthesis of vitamin B12 by the healthy gut flora. Furthermore, it is precisely through the one-sidedness of meat consumption without sufficient vitamin C that the absorption of iron is made harder and the digestion of meat, fish, eggs and dairy products consumes more calcium than these foods supply, even leading to an undersupply in the long term. Moreover, the ptomaine produced by the putrefactive bacteria considerably disrupts the functioning of the gut in the long term and the layer of hardened mucous, protein and various digestive remains on the gut walls, which are gradually getting thicker and thicker, make it harder and harder for the digestive system to send the needed nutrients from the gut to the body at all. The result is an undersupply on all levels. We literally starve sitting in front of full pots. We have, thus, identified what is actually to blame for malnutrition and have once more unmasked an alleged friend as a foe.

Contrary to all the fear-mongering, only a naturally varied vegetarian diet in the sense defined above gives any chance of absorbing all substances in the correct amounts and combinations our body requires for its functioning, and even more so for its development. When we see what indescribable riches simple nature has given us, it is a sign of abysmal ignorance to dismiss them as inferior, in the manner of the nobility in previous centuries, and rather keep to the pathogenic fleshpots and denatured industrial products. In contrast, let us take a brief look at plants that grow everywhere in abundance largely unnoticed but which are no longer considered to be food at all today or at best as food for poor people, but which remind us of the Hunza tribe or Thomas Parr, whom we encountered in the previous chapter: wild garlic, for example, contains just as much iron per kcal as parsley, our top-ranking food, and its calcium content surpasses our top scorer spinach by 100%. With 150 mg, sorrel contains equally as much protein per kcal as pork but, at the same time, also 199 µg of iron – that is 36 times as much as pork and even 16% more than parsley – and 3 mg of calcium, one hundred times the amount in pork. The stinging nettle is a truly incredible plant, breaking all records with its approximately 185 mg of protein per kcal, 20 mg of calcium – over 600 times as much as pork! – and 245 µg of iron. At the same time, it also provides over 10 mg of vitamin C per kcal, 8 times more than oranges. But the ubiquitous dandelion also scores excellently with its 60 mg of protein, 4.2 mg of calcium and 69 µg of iron per kcal in comparison with the so much praised – but pathogenic – animal foods.

Therefore, anyone who thinks they have problems with a wholefood vegetarian diet, it does not agree with them or does not taste good should, for the sake of their health, try even harder to get out of this state of degeneration. Unfortunately, we can get accustomed to so many things, also things that slowly but surely destroy us. But as soon as you have recognised that you should exert every effort of your will to get out of this ruinous process and back to the proper behaviour and mode of functioning, meaning – as we have now discovered in every detail – categorically giving up meat, fish, eggs, mushrooms and algae.

However, that is unfortunately not enough. We humans have over generations, in fact, thought out so much nonsense, which today pursues us like a downright curse and which we can only free ourselves from with the greatest difficulty – cigarettes, alcohol, drugs, refined sugar, white flour, refined fats and oils, taste enhancers, preservatives and many others. These intentionally designed and tuned creamy, crunchy or roasted tastes and oral feelings that do not exist in nature are for many people the last and often most important argument for not changing their diet. They need meat because vegetarian food does not have the same "bite." In other words, they are ready to sacrifice their health and even their lives for these fleeting illusions.

For the main part, this is based on ignorance, but even when they encounter truth most people willingly let themselves be convinced by the interested industrial branches or other lobbies, only so as not to have to change their dearly held habits. In this case, it is not, in fact, a question of having to do anything: it is only a matter of being aware of the consequences our own behaviour will have. The rest is subject to each individual's free will – without any ifs but also without any buts. Yet, the whole thing unfortunately becomes irresponsible and dangerous when it involves people who cannot simply act in accordance with their free will, such as children, or without being punished with ostracism and contempt from their social environment, as is the case with most of us. We see this problem most clearly with alcohol. Although everybody knows that alcohol alters and impairs normal bodily functions, leads to addiction and can ruin health and lives, consumption of alcohol is not only tolerated but even socially promoted. Thus, there is no celebration in politics, business, cultural and even in religious life that is not seen as an occasion for a good wine or a glass of champagne. And if someone does not want to join in, it is insinuated that they do not know how to celebrate, are a spoilsport or have a problem with the reason for the celebration. The person is then stamped as an outsider with comments that he is not a real man, a sissy or just not grown up yet or takes everything much too seriously. And all that is only because the person refuses to impair their health with a poison that is not banned simply because everyone, including those responsible, are addicted to it. Just imagine a similar situation with so-called hard drugs! But we can also find examples for them: in Bolivia the growing, sale and use of coca is completely legal above an altitude of 2000 m. Why? Because everyone there uses it.

The same mechanisms are also effective with smoking and food. Only when someone has to forgo something because of doctor's orders is it accepted by their environment without contradiction and with great sympathy. In contrast, not wanting to get ill is obviously still not a socially accepted argument. But we ARE all ill – with or without a doctor's certificate. We are miles away from true health and therefore we should no longer let ourselves be lulled into a false view of reality. Even if it is allegedly "only a little" or "only now and again", our society's state of health shows where our eating and consuming behaviour has led us and will go on leading us. Everyone should get aware of this and then set their priorities accordingly. In doing this, taste will be the smallest problem, even if it now appears so important to us. For whose first beer or first cigarette tasted good? Rather, how many attempts and efforts to get used to them were necessary to make it and belong to "normal society"! Today, the organs of taste have got used to them – unfortunately to our disadvantage. But shouldn't it be equally possible to readjust them to our advantage? Certainly – but only if it is important to us. That is a question of consciousness, of conscious being. For someone who has decided to themselves regain control of their life, their health, their future and hence their fate, nothing is impossible. Equipped with the right information, they will manage to bring their behaviour into harmony with the natural laws again and, in doing so, perhaps even give valuable impulses to those who made these changes so hard for them at the beginning. We would not be homo sapiens, the crown of creation, if we were to persevere in handling and using our bodies wrongly even when we have found the instructions for use again. At least, we should test them and not just for a few days. As the change takes time, a period of at least six months is indispensable. But then each one of us will know personally if they are correct or not.

Being conscious not only means enjoying lovely sunrises and sunsets or perceiving trifles that most people pass without noticing but also that everyone is aware of each of their own acts, their significance and the extent of their consequences. This includes knowledge, information and, above all, open-mindedness. At present, the situation is that we are pouring buckets of water into a barrel and are then surprised when it at some point "suddenly" overflows – because of a drop. That mainly happens out of ignorance but, to a greater and greater extent, because of stubbornness, lack of insight and unwillingness.

But it is important to become conscious that the consequences actually go far beyond health. For, as ignorance is no excuse with human laws, neither does ignorance or unconsciousness protect a person from consequences with natural laws. The universal law of cause and effect is, in fact, equally unerring but also equally relentless as any other natural law.

Why is it then that most of us are not conscious at all that the piece of meat we are just putting into our mouth was part of an animal that people have only reared and fed for the purpose of finally killing it, cutting it up and eating it? Why don't most people waiting in the queue at a butcher's or in the meat department of a supermarket think at all that everywhere there the products of a large industrial killing and destruction industry are being offered for sale – and consumption! –absolutely dwarfing Hitler's or Stalin's concentration camps, except that here it is not about humans but "only" animals? Do we really not know what we are doing, or do we perhaps think of it and still go on?

Part of us at least knows it – our inmost being, our soul. And it suffers because of it. For it knows that we torture, mistreat and kill living beings, our brothers in the animal realm, to satisfy our palate, for the sake of the bite. However, our body has got used to it and our mind is convinced it is right and necessary and so our soul has no chance of being listened to. And yet it knows – and suffers. We ought to at last start to face these emotions suppressed into our subconscious – for the sake of our own development, our own future and our own peace of mind. Instead, most people are afraid of the realisation and the truth and prefer to remain unconscious, to, in fact, absolutely close their consciousness and run into destruction with the majority. That is the more profound reason why our intellect thinks up all possible types of arguments, reasons and alibis to override the soul and not to let in the truth at all. Even the Bible, the foundation of an entire world religion, was "corrected" after the Council of Nicea in 325 AD to enable Constantine "the Great" to continue to indulge himself with meat and wine and still belong to Christianity at the same time. That is also the reason why many people react in an intimidated manner and wave the matter off as harmless or justify themselves almost aggressively, when they are asked about eating meat. And it is, finally, the reason for many mental problems, where the soul – as in Martha's case – expresses through the emotions that something fundamental is not in order.

Everybody is free in their actions – that cannot be emphasised often enough -, but everybody also has to take responsibility for them. At any rate, health is not attainable in this way, not even in today's common superficial sense. Therefore nobody should continue to cherish this unrealistic expectation. We will also only progress on the path to and the quest for true health when we have overcome this hurdle. So let's open ourselves to this information and implement it for at least six months in order to examine it through our experience. That will be a twofold test for us. For first we will test if a wholefood vegetarian diet really makes a difference and is in fact better. Secondly, we will also test whether our development and the search for a higher meaning in life are more important to us than our dearly held habits.

In doing so, we can – and should – additionally assist our mind, for in its current confusion it is like a computer caught in an endless loop. But we will speak about this in a later chapter. Now, we, first of all, want to explore other chapters of the lost instructions for use for our body.

5. A rolling stone gathers no moss

"Cross-country shoes? On the first floor, please, in the winter sports department." First of all, Klaus had to explain to the shop assistant that he wanted to walk and run, not ski. That was 1977 in Berlin. Although cross-country running is, to some extent, part of good German tradition, running was not customary anymore. It required a mega-boom in the USA to bring it back into fashion under the name of "jogging." This boom was already in full swing on the other side of the ocean at that time, after Dr. Kenneth Cooper had triggered it with his book "Aerobics" in 1968. Thus, at the end of the 1970's more than 25 million people were regularly on the streets running or jogging and, at the same time, the number of deaths from heart disease decreased by 14% within a decade – an impact generally assigned to the boom set off by Dr. Cooper.

Yet, this wave had not spilled over to Germany even in 1977, as the experience of Klaus Haetzel, head of the Senate Press Office, showed when he was just starting to be more interested in the sport of running. He started to run regularly and even to train intensively and two years later took part in his first marathon, which he, however, did not manage to finish. Then he was confronted with a diagnosis equivalent to a death sentence for many people still today, namely cancer or, more exactly, advanced cancer of the colon. He had to undergo an operation to remove a tumour as big as a child's fist together with part of his colon. Klaus did not want to let himself be got down by the disease and even less by radiotherapy or chemotherapy. On the contrary, he decided to simply run away from it. He resumed his running training already in hospital by dragging himself along the corridors and up and down the stairs. After his discharge he carried on with strict walking and, in this way, was able to increase his fitness slowly but surely. Only six months later, he ran a marathon again and this time finished it in less than 3½ hours and after that he ran wherever and whenever he could. There was no marathon he did not run until he shifted to triathlons three years later. He has, meanwhile, succeeded several times in doing the Ironman, a triathlon in which the participants have to first swim 3.8 km, then cycle 180 km and finally run 42 km in succession – and all that in a maximum of 17 hours. And what happened to his cancer? It fell by the wayside.

That is only one example of many cases in which people well and truly escape a life-threatening disease by demanding high performance from their body. In this way, they prove all their body is capable of, what forces it can mobilise, even when seriously malfunctioning, and that by doing so it is even able to heal life-threatening diseases. Yet, they most clearly show – as we will see in the next chapter – that what matters is our consciousness, on what our mind considers possible and what it decides to do. For unlike with Klaus, for many thousands of other people the diagnosis of "cancer" is a death sentence, which they themselves execute.

But let's come back to jogging, running and Dr. Cooper in America. Was that really all to his credit? Certainly not. He actually only picked up a quite elementary natural law of our body and applied it. But what was undoubtedly to his credit is the fact that he understood how to convince many people around the globe that this natural law is an indispensable part of the instructions for use for our body and that it brings health benefits across the board if we follow it. Like everything in nature, this natural law is very simple; it is in fact so simple that we take it for granted and consider it not worth mentioning. It says that our body is made for movement and all its mechanisms function all the better, the more demands are placed on them and the more they are trained. That indeed sounds like a platitude. And yet most people seem to be of the conviction that their body will always be fully available to them with all its functions, even if they sit the whole day, use their car to drive to the letter box on the next street corner and, in principle, always use the lift to get to higher floors. When the body then fulfils its tasks less and less well and fails or is overtaxed more and more often, we ascribe it to age or some inexplicable disease – but not to the fact that all its mechanisms are rusty. However, any owner of a machine which has not been used for a long time makes sure all its parts are oiled and cleaned before it is put into operation again. For sand in the works causes it to break down.

During his 13 years with the US air force, Dr. Cooper did extensive scientific research on more than 15,000 people into various physical exercises, proving so impressively that regular dynamic exercise has a positive impact on health, that this has been recognised and adopted worldwide by many millions of people and representatives of medical science. In addition, he introduced a points system, enabling every-body to determine and monitor the necessary amount of exercise they need. The foundation of this system is, however, questionable, as, firstly, it is based on an average of the social status quo and, secondly, is geared to a goal whose underlying criteria are not precisely defined. For what is "fitness" or "good shape" actually? Some people equate it with a slim body, others with a muscular one. Another definition says that fitness is the state of the body in which it can fulfil its tasks effectively and without unnecessary strain or fatigue. We see that here there are great differences, which certainly considerably influence the amount of exercise regarded as necessary for each individual.

So let's leave scientific guessing and go back to the level of natural laws, where we are sure to find universally valid answers. Firstly, it is surely clear to everyone that mobility and muscle activity decline if they are not trained. Those who have had a leg or an arm in plaster for a few weeks or had to stay in bed for a long time know this, at least from painful experience. Afterwards, mobility has shrunk to a minimum and strength has vanished as well. But then the original state can also be restored quite quickly through intensive use of the body mechanisms. This principle not only applies to joints, sinews and muscles but to all physical – and mental – mechanisms and even governs our entire development. Thus, for example, a small child only learns to see when there is something to see that the child also tries to see. Through these demands on the eyes, the optic nerves and the visual centre in the brain, the related mechanisms then develop in such a way that the outcome is correct seeing. If we permanently blindfold one of the baby's eyes in the first few months of its life – as has actually been done in experiments with kittens –, the eye remains blind or at least has impaired vision. The reason for this that the development of the related mechanisms can only take place during a specific stage of development. If this is not possible, it cannot be made up for later. A similar rule applies to all other of the body's mechanisms. A child has a longing – supported by the adults in its surroundings – to copy its environment, which gives it the necessary impulses to make efforts to challenge and train its body and mind. As positive as this principle is for our development, it can naturally be dangerous and negative as well when the environment – parental home, fellow beings, society – create adverse or even harmful ideals which the child also tries to imitate. It is likewise negative when there is a complete lack of specific impulses, for then the child will not carry out the development concerned.

That reminds us strongly of the subject of "normality," which we spoke about at the beginning. If nobody, in fact, considers some particular thing to be possible or achievable, nobody lives it, nobody aspires to it and it will actually not be realised. That is the point we are now at, wondering what is actually possible and realistic or what our body's normal features and capabilities actually are.

But let's return to our bodily mechanisms. If their functioning really depends on our use of them, it is quite concretely up to us how well, how reliably and how enduringly they work. In this respect, we not only have control over which mechanisms we train but also to what degree. The extent of their functional ability depends on this. Little children demonstrate this to us in an exemplary way: they are constantly occupied with trying everything – every movement, every ability, every skill – and always want to do their best. At some point or other, these impulses get lost and we adults do not strive for any new capabilities and do not even make use of those we have already acquired, so that they gradually waste away more and more. That in itself would not be so bad if we still had our ancestors' way of life, where all their physical mechanisms were made regular use of, alone through their daily activities. But today we "no longer need" to do all that, we have facilitated so many things through our technical achievements and possess so many mechanical helpers to do everything for us that we ourselves are literally rusting. This not only affects our muscles, which determine our strength and appearance, but also the otherwise unnoticed muscles, our blood circulation, our lymph circulation, our respiration, our metabolism, our senses, our glandular system, our internal organs, our sexual functions, our joints, our excretory organs, our nerve function – in short, really every single bodily mechanism.

But how are we to carry out this training and how do we determine the right amount? Let's begin with our muscles, for they are the parts of the body that are most frequently systematically trained. Here, there are various possibilities: first of all, you can simply repeatedly tense and relax them without moving them. These are the so-called isometric muscle contractions. In contrast, isotonic muscle contractions are those which generate movement. Both maintain or increase muscle strength and mass, depending on the intensity. These two factors are not, however, directly dependent on each other, i.e. large muscles may have less strength than small ones. For the crucial thing here is how many of the muscle fibres are used simultaneously in a contraction. Normally it is 65 – 70% at the most, which explains why in extreme situations, such as fear of death, unexpected reserves of strength suddenly become available.

Training our muscles first of all increases intermuscular coordination so that more fibres are made to contract simultaneously and only then, with more intensive training do the muscle fibres expand in width, resulting in an increase in muscle mass. But intermuscular coordination is a matter of the nerves and this explains an interesting – and at first sight astonishing – experiment recently carried out by the neurophysiologist Guang Yue of the Cleveland Clinic Foundation in Ohio. He gave 10 volunteers between 20 and 35 years of age instructions to imagine that they were training their biceps muscles very intensively five times a week. However, they were not allowed to tense their muscles themselves, which was controlled by the researchers by observing the electric impulses in the nerve cells of their arm muscles. The testees' biceps muscles were measured every two weeks and an increase in strength of 13.5% was found after only a few weeks and this was even maintained for three months after the end of the exercises. Here, we can clearly see how mind and body are connected and influence each other, although it is only a very rough and superficial effect. We will come back to this in connection with Ritam Samation.

Besides the simple contraction exercises just described, you can also train your muscles with dynamic movement as in running, swimming, cycling, rowing, etc. This kind of exercise has the characteristic that – when done for performance and stamina – it takes place with a high amount of oxygen, meaning it is connected with aerobic (i.e. taking place in the presence of oxygen) metabolic processes. This is the origin of the name "aerobics," which Dr. Cooper gave his book and, thus, a whole category of training methods. However, if you carry out such movements only slowly and for a short time (as in normal walking), only a small amount of oxygen is used. The same applies for short bursts of extreme intensity (such as sprinting or jumping), which do not allow a sufficient supply of oxygen. Here we speak of anaerobic (i.e. taking place without oxygen) metabolic processes. The crucial difference lies in the supply of energy to the muscle cells, for which there are, in principle, three possibilities: from fat, from carbohydrates (glycogen) or blood sugar (glucose). The most energy can be released from fat, for which process oxygen is, however, necessary. On the other hand, energy can be obtained the fastest from glucose and glycogen, namely both with and without oxygen. In the case of a normal, light strain the cells obtain their energy from blood sugar or fat deposits. If the load becomes heavier, more fat is burned as it contains twice as much energy as carbohydrates or sugar. If the load continues to increase, more glycogen is used as the oxygen requirement for this is lower for the same amount of energy. For this reason, it is the main supplier of energy in the case of a more intensive strain, but only as long as the supply lasts. Glycogen is also used when very strong and sudden bursts of energy are required, for which the blood is not able to provide sufficient oxygen. It is then converted into energy anaerobically, meaning without oxygen, a process which is, however, greatly restricted by the lactic acid created.

So what happens when a muscle is trained greatly depends on the type of training. With a medium level of training – whether in the form of not too strong, systematic contraction exercises or dynamic exercise – energy is provided by burning fat when the blood is supplied with sufficient oxygen. When the load is very great or the intensity of the exercise is high, the cells increasingly switch to burning glycogen and even finally catabolise it without oxygen in the case of extreme strains.

As already explained, the coordination of muscle fibres, in general, improves with training so that the strength of the muscle increases and its mass also grows after some time. As well as increasing muscle strength, regular intensive training has, above all, an influence on muscle metabolism. The threshold above which glycogen has to be burnt is raised higher and higher and likewise the threshold for anaerobic metabolism of glycogen. Trained cells also contain – even in a state of rest – a larger number of the enzymes they require for metabolising fat and glycogen and increase their fuel supplies as well. Furthermore, their ability to exploit the oxygen in the blood is enhanced, firstly by being able to obtain more oxygen from the blood and secondly by increasing the number of supply arteries. All this is also noticeable in a normal state, as the cells overall obtain more energy from fat than from blood sugar. In this way, there remains more blood sugar for the nerve cells and the brain, which anyhow obtain their energy exclusively in this manner. Moreover, an adequate supply of oxygen can be assured with less blood, which, in turn, relieves the cardiovascular system. Another effect is the increase in stamina, as the body does not have to resort to utilising its glycogen deposits so soon and uses the time-constrained anaerobic processes later, if at all.

Dr. Cooper provided evidence of the influence on fat metabolism in a simple, but very impressive experiment. He gave two groups of men – one well trained and the other untrained – three-quarters of a litre of cream for breakfast and nothing else. Then blood tests were done on them during the day at regular intervals. After the meal, an increased concentration of microscopic drops of fat was found in the blood of all of them. However, the blood in the trained group was clear again after only four hours, whereas it took the untrained men ten hours, as their fat metabolism in a normal state was considerably lower.

The higher fat metabolism will naturally also burn more old stores and deposits of fat and cholesterol if they are not constantly being replenished through food intake. With a healthy diet, the cleaning of the blood vessels can, thus, be considerably accelerated by regular dynamic exercise. We saw that clearly in the example of Eula in chapter 3.

We have, thus, come back to diet again in this topic as well. As fat actually plays such a large role as a supplier of energy, you might think it is important to eat a lot of fat. But, in fact, the contrary is true. For, firstly, the body has no problem in converting the carbohydrates in food into fat as needed and, secondly, the fat in food is mostly problematic or even harmful, unless it is a natural ingredient of fruits and vegetables. As soon as fat is extracted or oil produced – even when it is done in the gentlest way – the molecules are altered and then only in the rarest of cases have the same effect as those in unaltered foods. Animal fats are harmful in general as they are hard to digest, contain saturated fatty acids and therefore tend to clot. Furthermore, wrong fats provoke global functional disruptions in the entire body, as fatty acids partly also serve as structural parts of the cell membranes.

Animal proteins are likewise highly problematic for the body and should be eliminated from our diet, as they burden the body with their acidic products of metabolism, are a very poor source of energy and, in addition, – and that is important in particular in connection with dynamic exercise and sport – they use a lot of water and minerals for their excretion. For this reason, there is a much greater risk of dehydration with a protein-rich diet.

These facts will certainly surprise many people, for the opinion is still firmly anchored in the public consciousness that athletes and sportsmen and women require meat and dairy products at all costs, which is also underlined often enough by the official side – and naturally by the meat and dairy industries. Yet, if we look at active sportsmen and women, we find that the overwhelming majority of them primarily eat carbohydrates. Many even do completely without meat and fish, at least for a few weeks before their major competitions. Besides, there is an ever-growing list of strictly vegetarian sportsmen and women, some of whom are even vegans, i.e. they do not eat meat, fish, eggs or dairy products. The latter are far from being insignificant provincial athletes but, on the contrary, they include the greatest and most important people who really wrote sport history, such as the "flying Finn" Paavo Nurmi, who over a period of 12 years set 25 world records in long-distance running and won 9 Olympic medals, or Edwin Moses, a four-time world record holder and twice Olympic winner in the 400-metre hurdles race. Some of them only became vegetarians in the course of their careers, for example the six-time Swiss decathlon champion Beat Gähwiler, while others were almost lifelong vegetarians like Murray Rose, who set 15 world records in 400-metre and 1500-metre freestyle swimming and won four Olympic gold medals, one silver medal and a bronze medal. He became a vegetarian at the age of two and won his first three gold medals at the age of 17.

Another example is Sixto Linares, who set a world record in the 24-hour triathlon in 1985. He said he started eating a vegetarian diet in high school, experimented with eggs and dairy products for a while and then stopped eating all animal products. At that time, his parents were very concerned and even when he showed himself to be one of the fittest men in the world over the following 14 years, it was difficult to persuade them to abandon their misgivings about his meatless diet. In 1985, Linares broke the world record in the one-day triathlon by swimming 7.7 km, cycling 298 km and running 84 km within 24 hours – and all that without the animal products which allegedly provide so much energy. In the meantime, he has ceded his reputation as the fittest man in the world to Dave Scott, who won the hard ironman in Hawaii six times, in Japan twice, reached second place at the age of 40 and fifth place in the Hawaii ironman at the age of 42. He is a vegetarian as well.

It is interesting and, after all we have learned regarding diet so far, certainly no chance that the very athletes who were able to maintain their peak performances not only once or twice but over many years were vegetarians. Martina Navratilova, who is described as the greatest tennis player of all time with her 18 grand slams and nine Wimbledon wins, is a vegan. Likewise the "fastest man in the world", Carl Lewis, who won nine Olympic golds in the 100-metre and 200-metre running races, four times in the 100-metre hurdles race and 13 more golds in other international competitions. He himself reports that he had always eaten a lot of vegetables but since 1990 has completely gone without meat, even becoming a vegan. With four world records and his 65th successive win, the following year then became the best of his entire sports career, which he terminated in 1996 with a gold medal at the Olympic Games in Atlanta.

Yet, even when it is a question of sheer muscle mass, meat is not necessary in spite of all prejudices. This was proved very impressively by the vegetarian Bill Pearl, who won the title of "Mr. Universe" five times. It is even the case that a non-vegetarian diet involves considerable physical risks particularly for athletes and sportsmen and women. Although it is true that frequent and intensive exercise helps the body to get rid of many waste products of metabolism more quickly, "sand in the works" has a much greater and more negative impact in the case of high loads. Thus, for instance, the symptoms of wear and tear, which appear in athletes' joints after some years, are only partly due to the great strains on them. Another prime factor is rather the deposits of uric acid in their joints, which rub with every movement because of their sharp, crystalline structure until arthritis and arthrosis develop. Due to the extreme conditions of modern competitive sport, symptoms of wear and tear would of course also appear with a vegetarian diet, but with a healthy diet intense – even exceptionally intense – exercise is no problem for the body. The comparison with a machine which inevitably suffers wear and tear in the course of time is simply incorrect in this instance. For our body has a complicated and sophisticated system of lubricating, buffering and regenerating, which adjusts itself to any normal load and demands, thus guaranteeing unrestricted efficiency. However, if needle-sharp uric acid crystals deposit themselves in the joints, the best layer of cartilage, the best joint lubrication and all the synovial bursae in the world cannot prevent injuries occurring with every movement, so that at some point the body's ability to carry out repairs is overtaxed. If, in addition, the consistence of the lubricant is altered because of wrong ingredients in the diet and if the supply of nutrients and raw materials to the joint is made difficult or even prevented by deposits of animal protein, saturated fatty acids and cholesterol in the supply arteries, the problem can no longer be kept under control. In a similar way, changes in the cartilage structure also occur and these can have fatal consequences, above all for the intervertebral discs. For when these lose their elasticity and flexibility, they can slip out of position during normally harmless movements or even tear. This results in the increasingly frequent problems with slipped discs, the cause of which is not that people are making more and more acrobatic contortions but that they are training their supportive apparatus less and less and, at the same time, changing its structure with a wrong diet. If, in addition, there are uric acid crystals in the vicinity of the spinal cord, it becomes really dangerous. For then serious injuries of the nerve fibres may occur, leading to paralysis in an extreme case. Some people get a slight idea of such impairments of the nerve tissue in the form of lumbago or sciatica. In these cases, there is irritation and injury of the nerve tissue due to crystalline deposits, which mostly require a long period of complete rest for healing.

In the other tissues, uric acid deposits and hence rheumatic complaints with movements and strains of all types may sometimes arise as well. The arteries are other frequent places for deposits, which together with the thickening of the blood from saturated fatty acids and cholesterol have an extremely adverse effect on the efficiency and stamina of the muscles. For – as we saw before – an optimal blood supply is crucial in this respect. If this is not ensured, the cells have to switch to metabolising glycogen anaerobically sooner for want of oxygen, leading, after a relatively short time, to muscle pain and a loss of performance, due to the release of lactic acid and the using up of the stored glycogen. However, at the same time, the heart attempts to improve the supply of oxygen by increasing its pumping activity, resulting in a dangerous rise in blood pressure and pulse rate. If, in addition, the supply of the heart muscle with oxygen is impaired because of deposits, a fit of angina pectoris or even a heart attack may soon occur.

The body has similar problems with the necessary removal of heat created in the muscles. For good blood circulation is necessary to transport heat to the skin, where the evaporation of sweat generates the necessary cooling effect. However, if not all the cells are reached because of deposits in the arteries and thickened blood and, in addition, insulating layers of deposits have formed under the skin, the equalisation of body temperature is made extremely difficult. In its turn, the body attempts to equalise the temperature by increasing the heart beat and sweating more profusely, but it is only successful to a limited extent, while placing a considerable strain on the circulation.

The same problem arises with the removal of waste products of metabolism in the muscles.

These arterial deposits are made worse if we try to compensate for the dehydration and demineralisation of the body, due to the digestion and excretion of animal proteins, by drinking beverages containing minerals. For this replaces the body's own minerals with synthetic, foreign mineral substances, which mostly cannot fulfil the body's purposes and are likewise deposited. In this way, calcification in the truest sense of the word takes its course. Thus, not only physical attrition but also mental decline is not a normal phenomenon of aging but a degenerative consequence of an incorrect diet. Even baldness, which has become so normal for men in old age, is only due to the hair cells not being sufficiently supplied with nutrients and ceasing to function.

Therefore a person who wishes to have an attractive, well-proportioned body even at an advanced age, would do well not only to practise external body-building but, at the same time, to take care of the inner beauty and cleanliness of their body. Although we may not see this for a long time under normal conditions, it becomes very noticeable under great strain and with increasing age. In accordance with the ancient Greek principle "Mens sana in corpore sano – A sound mind in a sound body", it then ensures mental clarity and flexibility without signs of aging, even at an advanced age. To this end, however, any "rusting" must be avoided by not burdening the body with incorrect food and simultaneously training every part of the body and every bodily function adequately and regularly.

But what is adequate in this connection? And what is too much of a good thing? As always, our body itself gives us the answer. Thus, we have seen that it is, by nature, a system that likes and is dependent on movement. For our forebears, movement was an everyday, permanent accompaniment of life. Every search for food, water or a place to sleep was linked to dynamic movement. Likewise, everyone had to be constantly in a position to run away or climb away from a danger. Besides that, long distances were covered in the course of time, either due to the search for food, to the climate or to communication. In contrast, today everything is within our reach and for most procedures we do not even have to stand up or leave the house. If that is still necessary, we have created all technical means, such as lifts, conveyor belts, automatic garage doors and the car, so as to reduce movement to the absolute minimum. There are anyway scarcely any dangers we would have to run away from today – and that is a good thing, as we certainly would not manage it anymore. But we would manage it just as little if the life of one of our children depended on us sprinting some hundred metres to get help or to save it from something terrible. And such situations are still possible at any time despite all the technology, and have become even more likely in view of the innumerable new hazards and our increasingly impersonal society. Thus, in spite of everything, it is useful and appropriate – for the sake of our health and our physical preparedness – to orient ourselves, at least to some degree, towards the way of life of our forebears, who were certainly far more in harmony with the natural laws than are people today.

Accordingly, the right training programme consists of moving dynamically at least once a day so that we really sweat. There are unfortunately still some people who hold the opinion that one should not go as far as sweating. Thus, for example, representatives of conventional Ayurveda warn in all seriousness that toxins start circulating in the body through exercise generating sweat. But that is in fact a good thing! We want possible deposits to be released and eliminated. And for this we need dynamic movement and sweating without fail. For, firstly, the waste substances leave our body in our sweat and, secondly, the sweat glands and the body's whole temperature regulation have to be trained as well. Anyone who is afraid of sweating because they think their sweat does not smell good should sweat more for this very reason. For sweat only smells unpleasant when it is full of toxins. Once these substances have left our body – and no new ones are taken in –, our sweat no longer smells strong or even unpleasant at all. If we have eaten fruits, it will even have a pleasant smell from these. In this way, the necessary degree of dynamic movement has already been fixed, as it is, in fact, individual for each person. For everyone has a different point at which they really sweat, depending on the state of their metabolism, their circulation and their muscles – but this point is exactly right for each person without fail.

Likewise, our body also gives us an unmistakable signal when exercise threatens to become too much. That is, in fact, the moment we no longer get enough air with normal breathing through the nose and want to start breathing through the mouth. We saw previously that the supply of oxygen to the muscles is the limiting factor which determines our stamina and performance. So if we do not get enough air, we have reached the limit, beyond which either our muscles cannot produce sufficient energy, our blood cannot obtain enough fuel and oxygen anymore, circulation breaks down or several of these factors occur simultaneously. At any rate, that means unmistakably that we have to slow down or stop immediately. Then nothing can happen. The prerequisit is naturally that we generally breathe exclusively through the nose, which also is consistent with its natural function. With dynamic movement problems with the heart and circulation only arise when we exceed this limit given by nature, breathe through the mouth, thus overriding and invalidating any warning signals.

We have, thus, reached a very important element of the instructions for use for our body, namely correct breathing, where serious mistakes are unfortunately made almost everywhere today and particularly also in connection with physical exercise. If we consider our nose and the air passages leading from it to our lungs, we see that they are the ideal instrument for inhaling. For they contain innumerable little hairs to keep back foreign bodies and, including the sinuses, the air passage is long enough for the mucous membrane inside it to bring air continually up to the correct temperature and humidity for the lungs. In contrast, the mouth, which does not possess any of these facilities, is therefore only to be used for breathing in cases of emergency. This can be noticed by anyone who unconsciously breathes through their mouth for a long time at night and wakes up with a terrible dry feeling and a bad taste in the whole of their mouth and throat region. But, likewise, only the nose comes into question for exhaling, for which, at first sight, the features of the nose do not seem to be necessary. For the moist and warm air from the lungs leads to a warming and moistening of the mucous membrane of the nose so that it is optimally prepared for the next inhalation. In contrast, if we inhale through the nose and exhale through the mouth, this process cannot occur and the mucous membrane in the nasal passages cools and dries out more with every breath, creating hard mucous, which additionally impairs the cleansing function of nasal hairs. The warmth and humidity of the exhaled air is, thus, released in vain through the mouth. For this reason, correct breathing means that we generally inhale and exhale exclusively through the nose. This applies everywhere, in particular with dynamic movement and sport. But the most frequent mistakes are made in these very cases, not only leading to circulatory problems but also impairing the lungs, as the higher breathing frequency results in their being greatly confronted with too cool and dry – and possibly contaminated – air. The lungs already have enough to do with the toxins and metabolic waste which the body eliminates in the breathing air. But at this point another major error is frequently committed by holding this used air loaded with toxins in the lungs longer than necessary. Many people think that they enhance the exploitation of oxygen in the breathing air by pausing after inhaling before they exhale. But the metabolic exchange in the lungs only requires fractions of a second, so that air held in the lungs contains hardly any oxygen but, on the contrary, is loaded with the metabolic waste released by the body. However, the latter needs to leave the body at once and only after that is a pause appropriate. Empty lungs are in fact the normal state, which is only interrupted by inhaling and exhaling. The inhalation process is, thus, a reflex that takes place automatically at the precise moment the body requires oxygen again. In this way, in a relaxed state there may be longer breathing intervals, which are completely natural. But even when running flat stretches, well-trained runners have a relaxed breathing rhythm with long pauses after exhaling. That is the state where you could go on running forever – and actually can as well.

We have thus come back to dynamic exercise, namely the best and most natural – running. Of course, you can also move dynamically in other ways, such as swimming, cycling, cross-country skiing, rowing, etc. Yet, running is the best way for many reasons. Here, we do not mean lethargic, monotonous trotting on concrete roads but rather varied running over fields and farm tracks and through woods, uphill, downhill, on slopes to the right and left, more slowly, faster, etc. Firstly, hard, inflexible concrete and asphalt put an excessive strain on the joints and, secondly, when running in the wood on uneven ground, changing and varied demands are made on muscles and joints. This promotes overall flexibility, also of the upper body, when you have to bend to the side to avoid tree branches, squeeze between bushes, duck beneath branches which are hanging down or jump over ditches and tree trunks. Walking is a human's natural manner of locomotion and, hence, optimally adjusted to all its mechanisms. It promotes natural bowel movement (peristalsis) and, thus, is also an effective way of preventing constipation. As walking was by nature always a part of the search for food, it should ideally even be practised together with the cultivation of hunger. A short run with real hunger in your belly and then, bathed in sweat, a holy bath in clear, fresh water – there is no better way to prepare yourself for eating. And everyone can certainly imagine how good food tastes and how well it is digested after that. Anyone who has had this experience knows what real enjoyment of food is and that it has nothing to do with culinary delights for the taste-buds.

Running with its elastic movement also provides all the other inner organs with a beneficial and stimulating massage. The same applies to the spine and skeletal muscles, which can relax wonderfully with light, relaxed running. Besides this, the muscle activity gives momentum to the circulation of blood in the veins and the lymphatic flow, not only in the legs. If Gabriel, whom we met in chapter 1, had gone running regularly in the woods, he would not have got problems with his ears and the external, manual lymph drainage would not have been necessary. Likewise, there is no better means of keeping your nose unblocked than running. After just a few metres, your nose starts to run as well until it has got rid of all its mucous. Running, thus, not only has a positive effect on existing colds but is also a prophylactic measure to avoid getting a cold at all.

Just like other kinds of dynamic movement, running is, after all, also an invaluable benefit for the mind because of the stimulation of the blood circulation and the increased supply of oxygen to the entire body. For a well-supplied brain freed from waste can simply think better and, above all, leave well-worn paths more easily and find new directions of thought to pursue.

Overall, body and mind become more alert, more efficient and more flexible – an important step in maintaining and enhancing health and well-being. These facts have also been confirmed by a US government institution, the Center for Disease Control and Prevention, which published a report evaluating numerous results of several decades of research into the connection between physical activity and health. The main result was that people who are not usually physically active can enhance their health and well-being by becoming physically active regularly. The improvements to health are greater, the longer, more frequent and more intensive the physical activity is. One thing that the report clearly established was that more regular dynamic exercise leads to lower mortality, regardless of age. This finding is important for all those who do not want to begin with dynamic exercise because of their advanced age and poor health, for fear of a heart attack or circulatory collapse. The first point in the report looked into these very cases and clearly found that this concern is unfounded and the contrary is even the case – provided, of course, that one follows the recommendations and bodily feeling and does not attempt a marathon or an Olympic sprint from zero. Our heart muscle – the most important muscle in this connection – still has to be trained slowly at first, having to some extent been kept as it were in a plaster cast over decades and allowed to waste. The report states concretely that regular dynamic exercise reduces the death rate from cardiovascular disease and particularly from coronary heart disease. Furthermore, it prevents or lowers high blood pressure, reduces the risk of getting diabetes, cancer of the colon and depression, helps with weight control, building and maintaining of healthy bones, muscles and joints and promotes mental well-being.

Dynamic exercise alone is not, however, sufficient to keep the body in optimal condition. Another important factor is using, stretching and extending every mobile part of the body. Thus, ideally every muscle should not only be used daily but strained to its limits. The same applies for stretching it, and likewise our sinews and ligaments. Anyone who thinks they have enough strength and do not therefore need to train their muscles needs to be aware that a lot of muscles not only become weaker but, above all, shorter if they are not used enough. The result is the only too familiar stiffness, when you can no longer bend, squat or turn so well or perform other movements. In the case of imprudent movements or falls, this can even lead to serious injuries. Yet, for the sake of simplicity, age is then always made to blame for all that, but the real culprit is by no means time or our body – which would be equivalent to blaming the Creator for giving us a defective body –, but ourselves with our years of lethargy and laziness.

The optimal equipment for such stretching exercises is a climbing frame, on which you can climb to your heart's content every day, systematically and consciously using, tensing and stretching every muscle and fully challenging every sinew and every joint. Only when we exceed our limits more and more will we experience what our body is actually capable of. In contrast, if we are content with the status quo, we will stay with it and tend to regress, just as an inhabitant of the tropics is already very cold at 10°C and cannot imagine that it is possible to survive at all at temperatures below zero. However, if they move to such a climatic zone, their body will get used to the new conditions and they will soon no longer have difficulties with it. That this is far from being the utmost the human body is capable of is proved by Indian yogis who live naked in the Himalayas and do not, for example, measure the state of their development by how long they can hold out in the snow but to what distance around themselves they can make the snow melt when they sit naked on the ground.

For someone who does not have such climbing facilities, the yoga positions recommended by AyurVeda Ritam as the basic programme to be carried out daily, provide a good and practicable basis. They involve the most important muscles and sinews and train their flexibility in a fixed sequence of tension and relaxation. As well as that, however, everyone should also practise so-called everyday yoga, which consists in performing every movement in full consciousness to the end, i.e. to the limit of one's flexibility or capacity. That means, for example, that you do not simply bend down to pick up something from the floor but that you bend down consciously from your hips until you feel tension in the hollows of your knees, or that you do not merely stretch your arm upwards to take an object down from a shelf, but stretch yourself upwards consciously from your shoulder, exploiting the whole range of mobility. In addition, you can tense and let go any muscle isometrically, i.e. without moving it, at any time and any place or rotate your shoulders, head, hands or feet a few times, roll your eyes, massage your nose, eyes or ears, thus making the entire day into flexibility and suppleness training for the whole body. In AyurVeda Ritam this is called Svayamkarana (self-help or self-doing). The crucial thing about it is not to attempt some form of acrobatics, but to invigorate all mechanisms regularly and take them to their functional limits. In this way, everything retains its best functionality, which even slowly but steadily continues to be enhanced.

As effective as these exercises are, they are also simple at the same time. It is actually only necessary to stimulate our consciousness for our body. It is, in fact, impossible to become healthy if we only think about it in the gym for two hours twice a week and otherwise forget it or even mistreat it with wrong clothing and a lack of exercise. In contrast, we only get to know our body properly through more conscious treatment of it and develop a different – sounder – relationship to it. Most people are not at all conscious of where the muscles in their body are and what functions they fulfil. For example, our eyes are also surrounded by small muscles that move them and hold them, but at the same time deform the eyeball when they are tensed, thus causing faulty vision. If you learn to "get to" them, to consciously influence them and, above all, to relax them, you can improve and correct poor vision in a natural way without glasses. Most people are equally unaware that there are muscles in our body that we can control only a little or not at all with our will. In contrast, if we learn this, we can use them consciously, for example in the case of our pelvic floor musculature, which can have very positive and pleasant effects on our sexual functions.

For perfect functioning in the intention of the "inventor" not only the bodily mechanism is necessary but also proper control by the mind. We have, thus, already seen with muscle training that the neural coordination of the muscle fibres is of crucial importance for the strength actually available. Other examples are the experiences of people with amputated limbs. They mostly feel as if the limb concerned was still there and think they can move it. So it actually still exists on the level of mind and consciousness. In contrast, if the area of the brain responsible for a certain part of the body is damaged by an injury or a stroke, the control function is no longer possible. For the person affected it is as if the limb has been removed and replaced by a misshapen sack.

Here, we are broaching areas which we will treat in more detail in the next chapter, where we will see what a huge importance the mind possesses for our health and, above all, for our development and that Ritam Samation provides us with a technique to systematically and effectively train our mind-body system to function optimally. In this, relaxation and letting go play an important part. Many people are, in fact, of the opinion that physical training produces better results the longer and more intensively we practise it. If we were to train continually round the clock, we would have the best success. However, this is not the case. For, like all phenomena in nature, our body is also subject to the duality of rest and activity. Activity is indeed important to provide stimulation and impulses, as we have seen in the course of the present chapter. But rest and relaxation are equally important so that the body can implement the impulses. Muscle strength or muscle mass, additional arteries, increased stores of nutrients, increased lubrication of the joints and all the other desired and important effects of dynamic exercises are not, in fact, brought about during the exercise itself but in the resting phase afterwards. Therefore no muscle can grow if it is in continual use without having the opportunity to grow. The deeper relaxation is, the more effectively the bodily impulses are implemented. That is why optimal relaxation is also part of optimal training as well as optimal movement. But we will also go into that in more detail in the next chapter. There we will see at the same time that not only the mind is important for the functioning of the body but also the body for the mind. For the mental mechanisms depend decisively on having the proper physiological foundations. They, thus, require a perfectly functioning nervous system, which, in turn, is dependent on all other bodily mechanisms and systems. Therefore it is doubly important to keep everything in the body in good condition and to train it regularly. This even applies for mechanisms such as sweating, lubrication of the joints, the heart, the lungs, the inner organs, blood flow to the skin, the sensory organs and the sexual functions.

We have already seen in detail with dynamic exercise how we can train sweating, joint lubrication and the heart and lung functions. But how are we supposed to reach our inner organs? Fortunately our body helps us here with a wonderful mechanism – the reflexes. Besides their pure task of movement, our joints actually also simultaneously function as impulse-givers for the vegetative nervous system and all the metabolic functions. They virtually have built-in switches, which are activated when they are completely bent or stretched, then sending stimulating impulses to the entire body. This is another reason to practise the yoga positions and everyday yoga regularly as this not only directly stimulates the joints themselves but, indirectly, all bodily mechanisms. The feet are especially important in this connection. For the soles of the feet are densely sown with reflex zones, which interact mutually with all the organs of the body. These give us the possibility to stimulate organs and mechanisms not otherwise accessible to us, which constitutes the basis of foot reflexology massage, but particularly shows the importance of walking barefoot. Our body is so fantastically structured that, when we walk barefoot, stimulating impulses for all parts of the body are generated literally at every step.

Unfortunately, we make much too little use of this nowadays and accordingly our health is not what it should be. Therefore we should not fail to take off our shoes and socks whenever conceivably possible in any way and walk barefoot, if possible outdoors in nature on a natural surface. Our daily run in the woods offers the best opportunity – after a period of getting slowly accustomed to it. That will certainly sound rather strange to most people today – as we have been spoiled so much by our social standards! However, it was still not uncommon to go barefoot in the summer before and during World War II, which members of that generation will confirm. It was not until the post-war period that it became frowned upon to appear without shoes in the course of the new civilisational trends from America. Yet, at that time nobody was aware what a loss this step would mean for our health. In this respect, Pastor Kneipp had practised just the opposite not even one hundred years before. He made the degenerate ladies from the nobility take off their corsets, shoes and stockings and chased them barefoot over the fields wet with dew back to naturalness. And an old chronicle from the 16th century displayed in a museum village in Wendland states that "this winter even the last farmer put on shoes," showing what vitality and what healthy blood circulation ordinary people still had at that time. But their diet was also plain and meagre, whereas movement was many-sided and ample. With us today it is just the reverse and, accordingly, also the consequences.

In fact the natural barefoot shoes we were born with are the best footwear we can ever imagine. They are equipped with a dynamic suspension, sensors for temperature, humidity and quality of ground, a sophisticated differential profile with a grasping function and a sensitive, but robust leathery skin. Besides, they provide a direct reflex massage from Mother Nature at every step. Their only disadvantage is that we do not perceive them as chic and therefore do not use them. Instead, we force our feet into tight, unnatural footwear, where they sweat and atrophy – and with them our entire body. That is why everyone should practise walking barefoot again, first on soft grass or in the forest, but then more and more on harder ground. Over time, the soles of the feet will get accustomed to it and harden so that you will then be able to attempt longer distances as well. To be on the safe side, at the beginning you can take a pair of shoes with you in your rucksack when you go hiking. What was Thomas Parr's recommendation for a long life? "Keep your feet warm" – but not with shoes, but through exercise. He certainly must have known it!

In winter, when it is too cold for our untrained feet, we can resort to regularly stepping on pebbles, in alternating tubs of warm and cold water. In this way, we continue to get our foot reflexology massage and, besides that, a stimulating effect on the blood circulation through the alternating hot and cold footbaths. We should make use of this effect for our whole body by regularly taking alternating hot and cold baths or showers or going to the sauna and taking a cold bath after it. Such "holy" baths in clear, fresh water, if possible directly from a spring, are invaluable for cleansing the skin of waste products and, at the same time, also stimulate the bodily mechanisms regulating temperature. Thus, such a holy bath ought also to be a fixed part of our daily routine at the conclusion of any dynamic exercise, for freshening up in the morning or as physical preparation for the Samation. Yet, a cold shower is only a less valuable alternative in this regard.

At the end of this chapter, we finally come to the training of the sexual organs, which does not, however, mean that this is the least important part. For some people, it may be offensive to train in the area of sexuality and for others astonishing that there is supposed to be anything to train at all. However, concerning this it should be remembered that the sexual organs and the sexual functions are quite normal parts of our body and its mechanisms. And as the body is the temple of our soul, given to us by our Creator, there is nothing unnatural or even dirty about it – unless we make it so.

Just like any other part of the body, the sexual parts naturally require regular stimulation to be able to function optimally. Every mother who has just given birth can tell a painful story if she did not train the flexibility of her vagina for a birth without a tear of the perineum or did not prepare her nipples in time for her sucking baby. Besides, in particular, the demand for lust-generating or potency-enhancing means, which has been unbroken for centuries and becoming stronger and stronger in recent time, also shows that a considerable deficiency must exist here. In this respect, the best lust-generating and, at the same time, potency-enhancing means is an attractive partner and optimally functioning physiology. This includes acute sensory organs, sensitive skin free of deposits, an optimally functioning nervous system, a sound heart, normal unthickened blood, arteries free of deposits, normally functioning mucous and hormonal glands, optimal functioning of the muscles and parts of the body concerned and an undisrupted energetic metabolism in the entire body. All this can – and should – be improved by regular training. This training relates to the whole body, but also specially to the sexual functions and the parts of the body involved, with the rule applying that training should take place *every* day if possible. If a suitable partner is lacking, it is better to train alone than let the mechanisms dry up. This particularly applies to women, most of whom still consider it unseemly to touch themselves "immorally" on account of their education. But as they are the very ones who try to compensate for a deficit in this area through eating, they very soon get into a vicious circle, in which they do not get what they need from their partners, compensate for it by eating, thus becoming increasingly unattractive, so that the man has less and less desire to give her what they both need, which she, in turn, compensates for by eating, etc. until the mechanisms have completely dried up. At the same time, the unhealthy diet and the unhealthy lifestyle lead to him having erectile dysfunction more and more often or later permanently. But especially for post-menopausal women it would at last be possible to devote themselves to their sexuality without fear of becoming pregnant. But men in this age group are mostly not capable of having sex anymore.

Only regular training and a healthy life on all levels can lead people out of this vicious circle. This also includes getting to know your own body better and also your partner's. Thus, for example, a man and a woman can get much more out of sexual intercourse when they regularly train the muscles of their pelvic floor. In doing so, the woman gets control over the contraction or relaxation of her vagina and the man over the ejaculation of his semen. Although these muscles are usually described as "without function" in modern physiology, such an error would certainly be scarcely conceivable in the grandiose masterwork that our body is. Here, it is rather the concrete example of a bodily function, which, despite mentions in old writings, has been almost completely forgotten today. And as nobody lives it, nobody learns it and nobody is capable of doing it. But with men, it is similar with urination. If nobody told children they must not simply start peeing any time, nobody would learn to control their flow of urine and we would have another functionless muscle. In just the same way, men can learn to control their ejaculation, at last having an active influence on the prolongation of sexual intercourse as well and not only on interrupting it.

So here we have come back to the point where the crucial factor consists in what our mind considers possible and strives for. Therefore it is now time to look into the mind and its natural laws in more detail. In doing so, we will simultaneously find that completely new unexpected dimensions open up to us.

6. The thing about the mind

We already realised at several places in the previous part of this book that our mind holds a crucial key position in our attempt to uncover the secret of true health and find out how our body is actually supposed to work and what it was really created for. In fact, the mind plays such a central part even in simple everyday procedures – without our being conscious of it – that we must be constantly surprised that everything works so smoothly.

As a small example, let's consider a drive to the country with the family. In spite of the speed of the car, the driver always has a complete view of all the road signs, intersecting roads, oncoming traffic and the cars in the rear and side mirrors as well. At the same time, he brakes, changes gear and accelerates as necessary – without thinking about it. We become aware of what a feat this alone is if we think back to our driving school lessons, when every change of gear was an adventure, jumping and jolting and occasionally stalling the engine. But now everything just happens by the way. The driver even listens to the radio, talks to his wife, repeatedly tells off the children, who are arguing in the back seat, and reviews the unbearable discussion he had with his boss the previous day. All these procedures are subject to the activity of his mind. But that is far from being everything. For, at the same time, his mind is monitoring the digestion of his lunch, the proper distribution of nutrients, disposal of undesired metabolic waste, breathing, heartbeat, liver and kidney functions, the immune system, the function of the hormonal glands and their coordination with the emotions, is coordinating the healing of a finger the driver cut the previous evening and the cold that is still not quite gone and growth of the muscles stimulated by yesterday's training and, finally, the continual renewal and replacement processes of the body as well. All that – and a whole lot more we are not able to list here – constantly, simultaneously and without the slightest error!

But is that really true? Hadn't he just misunderstood something his wife said? And he had been darned late in noticing that car coming from the right a moment before! Besides that, he had physical stomach ache because of his stupid boss and his cold should have been gone a long time ago. In addition, we saw in chapter 3 that this exchange and renewal process does not work quite as it should. So something is probably not quite in order.

If we have another look at this impressive list of tasks and mentally add all those we have not mentioned here at all, a comparison suggests itself with a computer, which has too many programs open and sooner or later begins to "go haywire." This can express itself in some programs getting stuck so that they can no longer be executed, in a program getting caught in a loop and performing the same operation again and again without it being possible to stop it, or even making errors, i.e. executing different commands from those it has been given. At any rate, it gets slower, the performance per program declines, and if everything goes wrong, it stops and nothing more happens. We know what to do with a computer in such a case: we have to reboot it. There are even special key combinations and buttons for this. But what do we do with our mind?

Probably everyone has experienced cases of such breakdowns with programs getting stuck, and the long-term physical consequences of the mind being chronically overloaded are obvious enough everywhere. An example of an endless program loop was Herta, a middle-aged woman who came to a Ritam Samation course in a small rural community in Germany. She had attracted attention during my informative presentation, as she constantly jerked her head irregularly and uncontrolledly. She reported that she had had this problem since her youth and it had got worse and worse recently. She attended the course and after her first instructional Samation her jerking had already considerably lessened. During the course, she said that friends kept asking her in surprise what she had done to improve her issue so enormously. After about a month, she came back once more to express her thanks for the downright miraculous help. No more head jerking was to be seen.

"It only occurs sometimes when I am very agitated," she said, "but I will get rid of that as well."

Another miracle through AyurVeda Ritam? A computer novice will certainly have a similar impression when his computer crashes for the first time and a professional comes and reboots the computer with a seemingly magical key combination and after that everything works smoothly again. Even though this analogy may be simplified and certainly has many shortcomings, it is consistent with reality in many decisive points so that it enables us to better understand a whole range of mental processes. Thus, our mind is also caught in numerous loops and spirals and, on the other hand, cannot execute some of its programs, or at least not correctly, because we hold it permanently on the level of conscious thinking and overtax it. Neither it – nor we – are able to release it from this level, "shut it down" or "reboot" it. One person or another may succeed in "switching off" sporadically for a long or short time – which is always described as very pleasant and desirable – but at the crucial moment we lack the proper "key combination" to bring order back into our muddled program.

At this point, all kinds of techniques and methods are implemented to release the mind from its conscious level of thinking, enabling it to execute a "restart." All possible tricks and gimmicks are used to bring this about. The well-known autogenic training, for example, tries to trick the mind by influencing the body. The innumerable meditation techniques systematically use special music, visual effects, particular texts, citations or refrains to relax the mind and to lead to an improvement of the problem. Some attempt to simply switch off the mind, i.e. to stop thinking. And with their psychanalysis psychologists go a completely different way by making people rationally aware of their blockages, thus neutralising them. But it does not seem to be clear to all of them that these techniques especially rely on the conscious functions of the mind, which are overloaded and therefore do not work faultlessly. Moreover, it is a contradiction in itself to want to free the mind from the conscious level of thinking by occupying it on this very level through hearing, seeing, reciting, thinking, chanting, analysing or influencing the body. In our computer analogy, this would be equivalent to wanting to start another program in addition to the crashed program, supposedly to rectify the situation. These techniques may have a certain effect if the mind is working normally, but not when it is anyhow already overloaded. Apart from this, the effect would certainly not be to switch it off but only to occupy it pleasantly, though still remaining on the conscious level of thinking. The process of psychoanalysis aggravates the situation even more as it – in our analogy – repeatedly executes the operation where the computer crashed. In this way, it gets more and more entangled, instead of any kind of improvement being effected. All kinds of relaxation techniques are of equally little use in the case of an acute malfunction. For their intention is not a "reboot" but merely a shutting down of some programs. That is certainly a sensible and advisable step when the computer is working normally. But once the system has crashed, with an endless loop running somewhere or part of the memory no longer being available at all, the only thing that helps is shutting down and restarting the computer. We notice this at the latest when we want to go on working with the computer and the old problems are back again immediately.

We see that the mind's mode of functioning is obviously very largely not understood. Otherwise such useless or even absurd techniques would not come on to the market. Unfortunately, they have already succeeded in almost generally creating a completely wrong notion of the background information, because of their endless descriptions in the media and their glutting of the market.

For instance, Walter, an elderly gentleman around 60, attended a Ritam Samation course. He had serious physical problems and suffered almost continuous pain due to bone disease. But his greatest problem was that he was completely unable to switch off. He was continually preoccupied with brooding, reflecting, constructing, philosophising and suchlike and had properly spiralled himself into a mental world full of problems. However, already after his first Samation, his facial expression had visibly changed. He no longer made such a cramped impression and some deep wrinkles on his forehead had been distinctly smoothed. Although he himself was not aware of it, he confirmed that he somehow felt calmer.

In the first few weeks following the course, he contacted me several times a week and complained that he simply could not manage to meditate properly. In response to the question about what he meant by properly, he described his notions, which he had assimilated from some books or reports. He found it particularly bad that he regularly fell into a deep sleep after Samation and sometimes only woke up again after several hours. At no cost would he be convinced that this was, in fact, one success of the Samation, as he had normally complained of sleeping problems. During some meetings with him in person, I noticed that he looked much better than at the beginning, and he was much more relaxed during our conversations. Besides that, he himself reported that he had needed fewer painkillers recently. But he could not be dissuaded from his "failure" with Samation and actually stopped practising it after three months.

Here, we have a pitiable victim of the media before us or of people who talk about things they do not understand without having sufficient knowledge and, above all, without real experience of their own. Of course, it is nice to let gentle, meditative music wash over you with your eyes closed, while spreading pleasant scents of incense around the room, and concentrate on your breath, your solar plexus or your third eye, instead of permanently rotating around your futile everyday worries. But, unfortunately, that is just as superficial as when we shut down a few programs on a computer and start a nice screensaver. At that moment, it feels like a huge relief, but if, after practising this "relaxation technique" even for hours, you try to go on working with the computer, you realise that nothing has changed and the old problem is right back again.

Nothing should be said against all the manifold agreeable and beneficial relaxation techniques here. They are certainly important and useful in our hectic daily life. But it must be clear to everyone that they have nothing to do with real switching off, with genuine meditation or with Samation. A relaxing occupation and deep relaxation are simply two completely different things, just as wetting yourself by a lake and complete immersion are two quite different experiences, above all with quite different consequences.

In this regard, "meditation" and "Samation" are very similar in terms of the meaning of the words. The former comes from the Latin word for "middle", the latter from the Sanskrit word for "together". But what is today understood and practised unfortunately lies on two quite different levels. Thus, the so-called meditation techniques consist in drawing away or distracting the content of mental activity from the normal everyday content and orienting it towards other, more agreeable or more essential content – to the middle. In contrast, Samation takes the mind itself, not only its content, out of its normal everyday mode of functioning into the area of lower mental activity going as far as absolute rest. This difference probably becomes even clearer in our computer analogy. With "meditation" the computer stays in the normal area, only that nicer and more agreeable programs are opened instead of the usual programs. In contrast, with "Samation" the computer itself, i.e. its central processor, its main memory, etc. shut down so as to be able to restart from scratch.

I repeat once more that this is not supposed to be a degradation of meditation and relaxation techniques of any kind – however, only if it is a question of relaxation and occupying the mind with pleasant things. But these techniques are not suited to really switching off the mind and setting the related cleansing and regenerative processes in motion. For this, another level or another dimension must be brought into play, the experience of which has got completely lost in our everyday life. Some mystics and spiritual seekers from different cultures who dedicated their whole lives to this quest at some point or other managed to reach the level mentioned and were partly even able to reproduce this success on purpose. But even with many of them it did not get beyond a few ad hoc experiences, which they attempted to repeat throughout the rest of their lives. Nevertheless, these few moments were enough to profoundly alter their lives and their whole beings. So what can we expect if we enable our mind to access this level regularly!

A long time ago Thomas, a young student, called me and asked about the next Samation course. He had already read some books on meditation, had also tried out a lot of things from these books himself but now he really wanted to learn to meditate. He then came to the course, duly took part in everything but was very taciturn and did not comment anymore on his experience. After a good year he called me again and told me more about himself.

"I was very disappointed with Samation. After the instruction I went home and was really angry with myself. I still remember exactly how I repeatedly said to myself that you had really conned me. The experience I had in the course wasn't better or different from my own attempts out of the books. And the course wasn't exactly cheap. But then I decided to simply do the whole thing regularly and virtually subject it to a scientific test. I didn't want to make a final judgement after such a short experience. That would have been unscientific.

And now, two weeks ago, I had my second pre-degree exam. I had had the first one just before the course. That was a welcome test for me. And lo and behold, the two exams went quite differently. Not in terms of the results, but regarding my feeling and my state. This time, I was so confident and didn't have any trace of damp hands. In contrast, the time before I needed several handkerchiefs especially for my hands! And during the preparation for the exam I already had an interesting experience: in fact I had three attacks of sheer panic because time was running out and I saw that I wouldn't manage to finish everything in time. But then I simply sat down and samated and after that I was as cool as a cucumber and was able to learn productively and effectively for some hours longer."

In reply to the question as to how he had got on otherwise during the year, he continued to report:

"Actually very well. I changed my diet nine months ago and that has done me a lot of good."

"Why was that? And what is your diet like now?"

"Well, it was actually by chance. I was given a book and got stuck at the chapter about diet. What I read there shocked me so much that I immediately decided to change everything possible. The funny thing is that I went on reading a bit every day and then went on radically changing my diet every day. First I omitted meat, then eggs, then dairy products. Up to then, I had eaten in the student refectory. But when I read the chapter about cooking and seasoning, I never went there again. It was like an adventurous odyssey. First, I also had to make it clear to myself what I could eat at all and where I should get it from. After two weeks, I was, at any rate, a vegan raw foodist and, after that, I explored and discovered the world of food properly for the first time. A completely new world really opened up for me, a world of abundance, of infinite variety and fantastic physical experiences. However, in the course of time I also found out a few things that weren't correctly described or explained in the book and which then also caused me problems. But now I'm stable and I feel fantastic."

This example is deliberately described in somewhat more detail here as it shows several things in an impressive way. Thus, Thomas had read books and already had an idea about meditation and what it should feel like before the course as well. This is the reason he was also dis-"illusioned" after the course – rightly, for his illusion, created by himself, was gone. But luckily he did not make the same mistake as Walter, who projected his disillusionment on to Samation and thought it did not have any effect. Thomas allowed the possibility in his consciousness that he himself might have erred and that a different experience might be possible. He carried on and experienced very positive effects after some time. However, his perspective was also predetermined – as is the case with most people. For he considered his changed behaviour in the exam to be the epoch-making impact of Samation, while he did not connect it to the change in his diet at all. This was probably due to his first exam being part of the reason for doing the course at all. In contrast, diet had been no issue for him previously, but he nevertheless managed to make a complete turnaround within a few weeks, in a way that could not possibly have been more drastic and without any problems worth mentioning. He even found mistakes in the book on diet and was able to correct them for himself. Yet, if he had let himself be influenced by the predetermined ideas from his books and stopped doing Samation again, he would not have been able to experience all that. Walter and all others who decided as he did, therefore do not know at all – or do not even have an inkling about – what personal development they broke off for themselves.

The crucial criterium for judging Samation is, thus, not subjective experience while practising it but the impact afterwards, which mostly can even be assessed objectively. That, in turn, is like with the computer, whose restart is considered successful if everything works perfectly again, even if it rattled, clicked and blinked alarmingly during the shutdown and rebooting.

The same applies to Ritam Samation, or, more precisely, to its first part, Samarina. For when our mind has been released from its imprisonment on the conscious level of thinking and at last strives towards what it has been wishing to reach for an inconceivable time, namely absolute rest in its fundamental state free of any stimulation, it will realise that this is not quite so easy. Huge mountains of intellectual rubbish, emotional waste and informational trash have accumulated in the layers beneath normal everyday consciousness, making these areas so inaccessible to us that psychologists even speak of the "subconscious." On its way to the primal fundament, the mind will thus be confronted with all these impressions and deposits, which sets off considerable dynamics, also making itself felt on the conscious level, whether through thinking, emotional or physical processes. That is the reason why people often do not experience the deep, relaxing peace always described as characteristic when practising Samarina. On the other hand, this is an immeasurably valuable process, which, if practised regularly, clears up our consciousness and frees us from the old burdens that get in our way mentally again and again in the most impossible situations. There the reasons are, in fact, to be found as to why we, for instance, always react stroppily to the same kind of comment or get depressed, why we become anxious again and again in the same kind of situation or when we are reminded of particular childhood experiences or why we get along well with certain types of people, while never being able to get anywhere with others. Overall, this is the area which unconsciously controls and conditions us, making us unfree. When it has at last been cleared up, it is a huge relief and release, a downright renewal, in which we get to know ourselves properly for the first time and at last become what we really are – not what we have been manipulated into up to now by our subconscious old burdens.

In principle, this is the same goal that psychoanalysis also aims for. But unfortunately it goes about it in a completely wrong manner. It transports the old deposits out of the subconscious up into consciousness and deliberately looks into them again. Yet, in most cases this causes the same impression to be generated, thus intensifying instead of diminishing it. If someone, for instance, is dragging an unresolved shock around with them, it will not disappear by being experienced once more. Rather, the opposite is the case, quite apart from the fact that conscious preoccupation with old problems mostly clouds and confuses the present as well. What a lot of parent-child or partner relationships only really broke down when those involved made themselves fully aware of what had actually happened in the past!

That is why we should also especially here rely on the natural mechanisms of our mind-body system, which wash the old deposits out of us bit by bit, without our being concretely conscious of it. Only when they are gone do we notice that something has changed – like Thomas, who needed a new exam situation to realise that his fear of exams had vanished. In contrast, he did not realise at all how and when it had actually vanished and what was in fact the cause. The certain turbulence we described above as a concomitant phenomenon of the cleansing activity does not directly have anything to do with the impression the mind is just working on. Rather, it simply expresses itself in temporary increased thinking activity or sensitivity to noise with banal content.

Amidst all this clearing-up work, our mind still does reach its goal of primal stillness at its origin, but sometimes only for very brief moments, which nonetheless have such an intensive and enduring impact, which is almost indescribable. In these moments, it, in fact, reaches another level, enters a new dimension and gets into contact with the matrix, that global informational and structural field of infinite dimensions, which we will get to know in chapter 7. At the same time, there it is in its state of least excitation and in split seconds performs repair, regeneration and development operations on mind and body that it is not able to do in its normal state of everyday consciousness. This is the point of access to so-called miracle healings, to establishing the global balance of body, mind and environment, to true health. Yet, we unfortunately see that access to this level is largely blocked in our current state. That also explains why most people cannot even remember it anymore or at least have great difficulty in reaching it. We cannot simply expect it to be fully available to us immediately. First, we have to clear up our consciousness in regular, intensive painstaking work. In this, our mind is fortunately far superior to the mechanical computer. For when rebooted, the latter just switches off, empties its main memory and then starts again from scratch. Any wrongly saved bits of data on the hard drive or even programming errors in the operating system are not affected by this. In contrast, our mind works like a bottle brush and with every shutdown and reboot cleans a little bit more of the accumulated contamination, with larger and larger areas of our consciousness becoming accessible and available. It brings about an expansion of consciousness in the truest sense of the word, thus considerably increasing its own scope. At the same time, it is itself subjected to a reorientation through its contact with the matrix level, slowly but surely bringing its entire program structure into harmony with the natural laws structured in the matrix. But this – as with the bottle brush – requires regular practise of Samarina, the first part of Ritam Samation.

Apart from all its routine duties, the mind's task actually consists in helping us pursue our purpose and finding and achieving our goal. For this reason, it is permanently searching, immediately taking up new ideas, new impulses and new developments and in general wanting more and more and more … Today's technological and scientific advances, but also the flood of information and entertainment in the media, are a direct consequence of this innate tendency of the mind. Yet, all that unfortunately lies on the wrong level so that the mind cannot find what it is looking for and is therefore not more satisfied, but, on the contrary, increasingly restless. It is now even the case that our mind's activity has become perverted into almost the contrary of its actual task. Thus, it searches in completely wrong directions, which harm us more than benefit us, and has made itself the unrestricted commander of our emotional and bodily functions. It is the mind that determines what is good or bad, while our feeling and our physical impulses hardly have anything to say. We have already seen how its ideas about health, aging, proper diet and, in general, the correct handling of our body have become all determining. Therefore the human being is the only living being on Earth that follows its head in eating and drinking and moving, needs books to know how to have proper sex, does not rest when it is tired, but takes stimulating drugs, contaminates its nest with poisons and deliberately pollutes its breathing air with toxic smoke. Yet, it does not do all this to improve its situation but rather to its detriment. It systematically makes itself sick and old and, at the same time, also bites all the hands of nature that feed it. A clearer picture of complete confusion, overload and wrong orientation of our mind can only be drawn by having a look at the reality of our civilised societies. In this respect, self-programming is so strong that our mind is still convinced that everything is fundamentally correct. Although people look for relaxation or meditation techniques, it is not to make their mind at last capitulate and make a new start but to further reinforce and further it in the values and disciplines it has itself fixed, or so as to be able to overtax their bodies in even more self-destroying ways. For this, they use hypnosis and self-programming techniques to additionally stamp the patterns it has thought out on the anyway already misdirected mind.

How could it all get to this stage? And above all, how can we get out of it all again? We have already seen that a main element of the problem is the overloading of our mind. Already as a young child or sometimes even earlier, the mind is confronted with experiences it cannot digest and stores as impressions – either positive or negative. In addition, there is the inundation with impulses and information, for the processing of which normal sleep is inadequate and which thus amass on the mountain of deposits. In this way, a downright vicious circle comes into being. For the more our consciousness is filled with such impressions, the more the normal functioning of the mind and also of the body is impaired. Sleep becomes poorer and poorer and thus can process less and less intellectually and the body no longer provides the necessary physiological basis but, due to its own malfunctioning, even constitutes an additional strain on the mind. As with the computer, this, in the end, inevitably leads to a crash, which expresses itself at a different place in each individual. But, unlike with the computer, the system rarely simply stands still. It goes on working, but only with a fraction of its resources or with more or less obvious faults. With Herta, her tic was obvious to everyone and that is why she sought help. But what a lot of people walk around with similar or more serious tics, which are, however, not so visible, without it occurring to them that they need and should seek help!

Here, a second factor adds to the problem, namely our inner programming – in our computer analogy, our operating system. This basic program has been shaped by many generations and existences, countless human encounters, opinions, pictures, books, films, experiences, wishes, ideals, in fact everything that has entered our consciousness in some way. That is why it is based on so many basically contradictory elements that it is in itself highly paradoxical and hard to penetrate. In most cases, it has even become self-destroying nowadays. In this operating system, we have programmed what is normal for us and what is right or wrong. And our system works so accurately that all this is also implemented exactly. For instance, it is "normal" to go downhill after our mid-thirties, to be regular doctor's patients after the age of 40, to undergo operations from 50 onwards and to start dying after 60. It is likewise "normal" for physical performance, strength, mobility and fitness to decline with increasing age and for the mind to degrade considerably as well. In contrast, it is "abnormal" to think that one can fundamentally change anything concerning these facts through different behaviour. And it is certainly "wrong" to want a meatless diet, for then many necessary substances would be lacking. This programming is so strong that the mind actually even filters out news and information in accordance with it. Everything that confirms the program is a reinforcement and it just does not listen to anything that is in conflict with it. However, if the "anti"-information is too strong to be simply overlooked it is even frequently made into a bogeyman only to protect one's own basic program. How often real innovators first had to die at the stake for this reason in the history of humanity before their discoveries were written on their memorials as right and ground-breaking in the following generation!

Here we have come back to the starting point of our exploration, but from a completely different point of view. For here the question arises as to whether we would really recognise and accept answers to our search, indications of true health and the path to get to it or whether we would discuss them away with some alibis and deny them just so as not to put our operating system at risk. For it cannot be otherwise than that the answers we are seeking will be in conflict with our basic program. Otherwise we would achieve true health with our programming and would not need to search for it. With the question about correct diet, particularly the problems of meat, fish, eggs, mushrooms and algae, we already recognised how profoundly and inexorably we have been marked by our wrong behaviour up to now and want to hold on to it whatever it costs. Therefore it must be clear to us that we are running the acute risk of sacrificing our development to our present operating system. In this way, we even prevent ourselves from experiencing what actually lies in front of us, which would be possible and attainable.

How absurd this attitude is may be illustrated by a small – if not quite realistic – analogy. Let's assume for a moment that the common interpretation of life expectancy is actually right – in contrast to what we found out in chapter 3, i.e. that people really only reach the calculated age. Let's assume we are living in a distant Stone Age civilisation, where average life expectancy is only 13 years and everyone dies at the age of 13. For these people, puberty is thus the highest state of development, as there is nothing more for them. If someone were to come and tell them that it is quite different in reality and that a human being can live to 60 or 70 and develop much further and also were to tell them how that can be achieved, would they believe him and implement his information? Or would they perhaps rather laugh at him and chase him away, because what he said was in absolute conflict with their basic program?

Wouldn't we today also call anyone crazy who claimed that human beings can live several hundred years or even longer in the best of health and with mental clarity, even in natural possession of capabilities that we consider possible at the most for founders of religions and then only when we have nailed them to the cross? But, at the same time, our mind is in search of more, of a way out of our restrictive deficiencies and ought to accept any such information with joy and implement it at once or at least submit it to a test. But our mind is not capable of doing that as long as it is still under the influence of its extreme misprogramming and, at the same time, is on the verge of collapsing due to its self-made overload. Nevertheless there are repeatedly impressive examples showing what is possible when we just free ourselves a little from our basic programming and open ourselves to the regulative influence of the natural laws. Thus, for instance, Klaus was saved by programming his mind fully on exercise, running and the marathon. This meant that his focus was on fitness, performance, physical improvement and not on sickness, suffering, medicine, etc. We have seen the consequences: his body eliminated disease and achieved an unsuspected degree of strength and stamina.

In this connection, I recall a conversation with Samuk Deda which has remained very firmly anchored in my consciousness. We were sitting in front of his little house on a mountain in the Balkans. It was a warm, sunny summer day and Samuk's children were all playing in the field in front of the house. His second oldest son G. was doing a training session with his smaller brothers and sisters and was just demonstrating a flip-flop from a standing position. It was impressive to see his well-proportioned muscular body shining in the sun.

Then Samuk said, probably more to himself than to me:

"You can hardly imagine that G. had polio!"

I thought I had not heard correctly. And, as if to show the absurdity

of this statement, G. was performing a back handspring from a standing position just at that moment.

"Did I hear correctly? Polio?"

"Yes, it was terrible! The little boy didn't move a millimetre from me
for four weeks. He only wanted skin contact, nothing but skin contact
... and sweated incredible amounts. I didn't do anything the whole
time besides sleep and Samation with him on my chest."

"And the consequences?"

"Nothing, as you can see! Until a few years ago he was sensitive
to great mental strain. Then he got a slight headache and in the case
of great stress his legs gave way now and again. But now all that has
gone."

"How did you know what to do?"

"His body knew it. I only obeyed and with the Samation I created
order in the atmosphere."

"Why didn't you have him vaccinated?"

"You ask that?"

He looked at me in astonishment and then gave me a long lecture
on vaccinations, concluding with the following words:

"Vaccinations are a huge burden for the immune system and mostly
do more harm than good, particularly in small children. Above all, the
preservatives for the vaccines are absolute neurotoxins, which severely curb many children's mental development, also leading to serious
learning and concentration problems. You know what mental capac-
ities G. has today. He would hardly have had them if he had been
vaccinated as a child."

"Wouldn't that be a new therapeutic approach for polio that ought
to be published?" I asked him at the end.

"Thomas, don't forget that we have been living in harmony with
the natural laws and the knowledge for decades. Only for that reason
did his body and his mind have the ability to overcome the disease.
That is the actual therapeutic approach. Until that is in place, anything else is only a danger. You can't climb the twentieth rung of a
ladder before the first."

He was right. And as the first rung is obviously the most difficult for
most people, they declare the whole ladder to be an unrealistic fantasy
instead."

And so we have got back to our basic programming and have
learnt about another component, about which similarly fierce wars are

waged as about eating meat, namely vaccinations. Although, apart from a few exceptions, there are no statistics to confirm the repeatedly depicted great success of nation-wide vaccinations with many statistics even refuting it, and although more and more cases of damage from vaccinations have been revealed and the number of opponents of vaccinations is continually growing, vaccination is for most people an indispensable basic part of our health system, which must not be shaken under any circumstances.

Here, we have before us an example of a consciousness virus, such as is to be found in large numbers in our basic program. As in the computer world, these viruses spread like an epidemic from consciousness to consciousness and establish themselves everywhere mostly unconsciously. The whole of our society even lives from such consciousness viruses, for, after all, they are what determine buying behaviour, voting decisions or similar acts. Basically, we are no longer ourselves at all, but our mind carries out program commands which we ourselves do not want at all, neither have programmed, but which have, nevertheless, got a foothold in the form of a virus, resisting any attempt at reprogramming, while even going as far as self-destruction. We see this, for instance, in anorexics, who are still programmed to lose weight even when dangerously underweight and thus literally starve to death. But we do not have to fall back on such extreme examples: what a lot of people want to lose weight or change their diet and do not manage it because other elements of their basic program run counter to it! What a lot of people would like to stop drinking or smoking and do not manage it, although they know exactly what it means for their health! What a lot of New Year or birthday resolutions originate from such knowledge but then fail miserably at the first attempts to put them into practice!

And another example – what a lot of children do not like the strawberries from their own garden anymore because they do not taste like what they know from their favourite fruit yoghurt! We see how diverse these consciousness viruses and the related misprogramming can be. However, they all have one thing in common: they are not in harmony with the natural laws and manipulate us in this very same direction.

Now that we have elucidated most clearly where the causes and mechanisms of the colossal confusion of our mind lie, we want to turn to concrete help in finding the way out of these vicious circles. In this, our analogy with the computer can provide us with valuable pointers to a certain degree. We have already seen that the first thing necessary is to reboot the computer or release the mind from the level of conscious thinking to the level of absolute rest. That is actually only a release, a letting go, for the mind is by nature in search of more, something greater, something more fulfilling. Therefore it does not need to be enticed or pushed to the level of its origin, it goes there freely on its own – if it is released from the level of its conscious everyday activity. This letting go is the key, and we have already seen that almost all approaches fail here. In its first part, Samarina, Ritam Samation uses special word-sounds attuned to the current physical and mental state of each individual. In this way, everyone gets a key appropriate to their present constitution and this releases the mind from its conscious level of thinking and helps it to sink into contemplation.

We have already described figuratively what happens in this process. But also the objective methods of experimental psychology have made impressive findings concerning this subject in recent years. First and foremost we must mention the ground-breaking work of Professor Jacobo Grinberg, who unfortunately vanished in a mysterious and as yet unexplained manner in 1994. He showed in a complex, large-scale series of tests that the brainwaves in a meditative state differ distinctly from those in a normal waking state. They are more coherent, more orderly and more harmonious. Other vibrational patterns occur and other frequencies are involved. He proved unequivocally that these changes are more rapid and more marked, the more experience the person concerned has with meditative states. In other words, this means that the longer someone practises Ritam Samation, the more intensive the impact is, which is exactly consistent with the subjective experience we described previously in the image of the bottle brush. More and more deposits and obstructions are dissolved and the inward path becomes broader and easier. Seen physiologically, this becomes manifest in a restructuring of the brain, favouring a different mode of functioning with altered brainwave patterns. Besides that, Professor Grinberg and his colleagues at various universities found that in a meditative state distinct physical reactions are also to be perceived. Thus, the heart and breathing frequencies decrease, skin resistance increases and even the composition of the blood itself changes. Overall, these values resemble those of a person in a deep sleep but go considerably beyond them. The conclusion is that in a state of deep meditation the body is in an even more profound rest than in a deep sleep. This is indeed astonishing, for subjectively one does not feel it like that. Although you feel deep peace and relaxation, you are fully conscious the whole time. You perceive everything going on around you but do not register it because you are on a different level. Yet, as soon as you open your eyes and stop using the word-sound, you are present again. So there is no reason for the concern which is often expressed that you "dive down into something," from which you never return.

However, Professor Grinberg's results go even further. Stimulated by the coherence found in the brain and between the two halves of the brain and by subjective experiences of shamans and meditation gurus, he also made experiments with several people at the same time. In these he found that a person in a state of deep meditation influenced the brainwaves of another person even in a different room out of a Faraday cage. In other words, when we practise Ritam Samation, we not only create order and coherence in ourselves but also around us. That reminds us of Samuk Deda's words that he created "order in the atmosphere" through Samation when his son was sick.

But let's return to our helpless mind. Once we have removed some of the old unprocessed rubbish from our consciousness with Sama-rina, we have unfortunately not yet finished our work. For these im-pressions in our consciousness also had a physiological equivalent in the form of misdirected hormones or deposits in the nervous system. Although these substances have now been released, they are still in the body, where they are circulating around somewhere in the blood. So if we do not now ensure that they are completely eliminated, the cleansing by Samarina will be incomplete. This task is now assumed by Samaya, the second part of Ritam Samation. By means of a sim-ple, but extremely important procedure it serves to take the released waste to the excretory organs, thus effectively concluding the cleans-ing. All other techniques fail at this point, as they leave it to chance if any released substances leave the body or deposit themselves some-where again, only to wait until their next release to cause physical or mental problems once again.

At this point we see quite concretely how closely body and mind are connected in both directions. Every emotion and every mental im-pulse are directly implemented by the production and release of a par-ticular hormone or the activity of special nerve cells. But, conversely, infiltrated or released hormones or induced stimulation of the nerves trigger clearly defined emotions and mental activity. In this way, we can understand mood swings which actually do not have any external cause but, nevertheless, occur unmistakably. Particularly women are only all too familiar with this in connection with their monthly cycle. This is why everything we have found out about the body so far is simultaneously of crucial importance for the mind. For when the body is groaning under a wrong diet, lack of exercise or sickness, it also directly affects the mind. Everyone who wakes up in the morning with a headache or acute stomach ache knows this from their own experience. In this state mental excursions or emotional highs are not possible however great our wish or effort may be. For this reason, we are no longer surprised by the conclusion of the American report from the last chapter that regular intensive dynamic exercise increases mental well-being. For when the brain is better supplied with blood, the blood provides more oxygen and glucose and more toxins are eliminated in sweat, the nervous system can work better and the mind has quite a different basis for its activity.

Sleep is of equally great importance. For it is actually by nature the relief and rehabilitating mechanism for the mind and at the same time the regenerative mechanism for the body. But in order to be able to perform all these tasks, it needs certain indispensable conditions, which we are far from giving it. Everything in nature is structured in an alternation of rest and activity, for which day and night were also created. And when people still went to bed with the hens and got up with them, they were actually much healthier and more able-bodied. But today we have got used to making night into day, which even goes as far as seriously believing we are night people. Yet, that is nothing more than another example of the misprogramming of our consciousness. There are neither day nor night people, but only such who live in harmony with the natural laws and those who break them. In this respect, it is also of little use to stay in bed longer the next morning to get the necessary hours of sleep. For not every time is equally well suited to sleeping. Popular wisdom has from ancient times spoken of the value of sleep before midnight and AyurVeda Ritam speaks even more precisely of sleep before 10 pm. It is actually so – and everyone can find that out for themselves – that sleep has a different quality when you go to bed before and not after 10 pm. Of course, the so-called night people have to test it for a longer time, for they will probably not be able to fall asleep so early the first time.

But unfortunately there are even more serious mistakes with which we make the sound, regenerating sleep we so badly need impossible. Besides the bed itself, the mattress, the quilt, the pillow, we should mention the sleeping direction, sources of voltage or radiation from antennae in the bedroom as well as eating heavy food, eating too late or indigestible mental activity before going to bed. Unfortunately it would go too far to go into all the points mentioned in more detail here. We therefore refer the reader to the literature dealing with these topics in depth. But it cannot be emphasised too much how important sleep is for our physical and mental health. Therefore we should give it high priority in our daily routine instead of reducing it to a minimum. Unfortunately there are often people who are interested in meditation so as to be able to reduce their need for sleep. For them sleep is nothing but an unnecessary and undesirable waste of time. But that is a great mistake. For nothing works without the necessary rest, either physically or mentally. And it is not surprising that one of the first effects of Ritam Samation only too often consists in people falling asleep during Samarina or Samaya. The moment the mind gives up its programmed notions, leaving itself to be guided by nature, the body procures what it needs, thus replenishing its years of deficits. Yet, that should be the signal to the mind to sleep more in general so that Ritam Samation can carry out its valuable clearing work in consciousness optimally instead of having to serve as a pure sleeping pill.

So our own behaviour gives us control over what impact Samation has and what its goals are. Samarina and Samaya thus continually carry out important regeneration, repairs and further developments on physical and mental levels. Through its contact with the matrix and the related deep relaxation, the mind simultaneously also receives valuable impulses. Nevertheless, we still have our free will and can ourselves decide how and for what we use it all. Thus we might stay with our mistakes and vices just because of Ritam Samation, as they are ironed out again for the most part with every Samation. But, at the same time, it must be clear to us that then the entire or main strength of Samation will be used to neutralise the metabolic waste from our incorrect diet, the harmful effects of cigarettes and alcohol and other environmental contamination and stress, etc. – if it manages all that at all – and then nothing or only very little is left for any form of further development. So anyone who wants or expects more, must not rely on the "miracle pill" of Ritam Samation but must, at the same time, create and continually improve the requirements for this through changes in their own behaviour.

The optimal and most effective way to develop further is, accordingly, parallel approaches on physical and mental levels. A correct diet and intensive physical exercise thus create the requirements for Ritam

Samation to have the best possible effect and being able to press ahead with regeneration, repair and further development, instead of having to struggle with the constant routine contamination. At the same time, Ritam Samation, for its part, creates the requirements for an easier change of diet, so that instead of a feeling of restriction and sacrifice one of benefit and fulfilment prevails, our weaker self does not thwart our good resolutions so often and any physical training is supported by the correct mental processes and, above all, by the necessary relaxation. In this way, the physical and mental levels mutually help each other to get from one step to the next and the entire development very soon gains its own momentum so that we anyway do not wish to go back anymore and instead are increasingly fascinated and interested to see everything that is going to happen.

Naturally, Samation should then also keep pace with the development that has been set in motion and Ritam Samation is indeed a continuous process, which is adjusted to individual development with so-called Sampranchas at regular intervals. This takes stock of the current state of development each time and adjusts the word-sound accordingly.

Now this may surprise those who have already concerned themselves with conventional Ayurveda and its theory of constitutions. According to this, every individual has a basic constitution fixed at birth, which cannot be changed and to which all the methods of conventional Ayurveda are tailored. However, this view is only a variant of the widespread consciousness virus, which is circulating in a similar form with regard to genes. In reality, nothing in our body or mind is, in fact, unalterable in principle. We have unfortunately proved this ourselves in a negative direction in the course of past generations and centuries, where one degeneration previously considered impossible after the other has become manifest. But the same also applies in a positive direction. Only we first have to create the necessary requirements and fundaments for it. If our genes or constitution were actually not alterable, where do the increasingly frequently occurring congenital diseases or the more and more chaotic constitutional degeneration come from? This incomprehensible myth is, however, unfortunately very frequently given as a reason for not changing anything in one's behaviour, since the problems are hereditary anyway. In this respect, just the opposite is appropriate. For here it is crucial to understand that, particularly in the case of congenital or constitutional problems, it is important to take countermeasures. An inborn weakness does not necessarily also emerge when we behave accordingly. But if we do nothing or even support the weakness, it is bound to break out, in fact worse and sooner than in other people. A congenital weakness is, thus, not carte blanche for wrong behaviour, but, on the contrary, a downright obligation to behave correctly so the weakness does not make its appearance and is not passed on to the next generation either.

So it is not only possible but even necessary to change our genes and our basic constitution to reverse all the harm our forebears and we ourselves have done.

That is also exactly one main effect of Ritam Samation, where the mind receives such regulatory impulses from its contact with the matrix that it is able to restructure the whole body. After all, the matrix is the global informational and structural field of creation, constituting the foundation of the whole universe with its living and inanimate nature like a mould. And our mind is the universal coordinator and operator of all our bodily processes, which it even – as we saw in chapter 3 – renews every year from scratch. If it is then freed from its overload and malfunctioning through the regular practice of Ritam Samation and, at the same time, slowly but surely brings its basic program back into harmony with the global system of natural laws through its contact with the matrix, things happen in our system that are, in fact, not normal in today's society but, nevertheless, more real than all the consciousness viruses which control us. How are the 13-year-old pubertal Stone Age inhabitants to learn whether anything else is possible in life beyond puberty, except by trying to reach it? And how are we to learn whether there may be a second – perhaps mental – puberty, which we will not reach at all or even torpedo with our present lifestyle, like women who sabotage their menopause by taking artificial hormones for fear of a calcium deficiency, which they themselves cause through their incorrect diet?

We mentioned at the beginning of the book that most of our genes are even today still unintelligible to our researchers. It is the same with our brain, for which we have still only been able to assign functions to a few individual sectors. Here, we are light years away from an understanding of it. But this is the very point where we have to begin, not through laborious and endless analytic research, but by following the natural laws and working towards a possible quantum leap, as has repeatedly been exemplified in the lives of single individuals in human history in all cultures. Here, it also has to be clear to us in principle that the mind does not only consist of intellect, and an expansion of our consciousness is not equivalent to an improvement in our intellectual capacity. An enhancement of our mental potential will not only lead to us becoming better at mental arithmetic or comprehending Einstein's theory of relativity, but, in addition, completely new dimensions will open up that are still more unimaginable to us than a modern adult was to the 13-year-old pubertal Stone Age inhabitant. So let's go the way of unfalsified nature, whether we believe in it or not, and we will personally experience that a lot will change, not only our constitution. In the end, there is no other way, for what else are we to orient ourselves by, in view of the present devastating "normality"?

Ritam Samation, at any rate, helps us in the manner already described to manage as well as possible on this path. At the same time, it is itself individually adjusted to the ongoing development by means of the Sampranchas, so that the whole process progresses in an optimal manner. After a year of regularly practising Samarina and Samaya, we proceed to the third part, Samshobha, which systematically starts at the point where a computer user one day goes to get a new operating system. For unlike our mind, the computer operating system does not change by itself. That is why the bugs remain in spite of regular rebooting, repeatedly causing the same problems – until the user switches to a new version, in which at least some of the bugs have been remedied. During the practice of Samshobha the mind emits impulses in an exactly structured alternation of deep rest and conscious activity, so-called Manas, which eliminate misprogramming by the resonance principle and then carry out reprogramming. These Manas do not have the goal of realising any wishes or desired patterns of behaviour but simply express fundamental natural functional principles, activating these simultaneously on the vibrational, intellectual and emotional levels. Samshobha thus differs fundamentally from techniques such as hypnosis, mental training or positive thinking, which operate on the level of our everyday consciousness and so only have available to them the effectiveness possible there. In other words, these techniques do not rewrite the basic program but only use it to execute additional program elements. But if the basic program already has problems, these additional elements are of no help but rather complicate things further. In contrast, Samshobha expands and improves the basic program, providing the mind with a better framework for its programs. In this process, additional Manas are assigned at greater intervals according to an ongoing principle, thus resulting in a strict adjustment to individual development.

Of course, there are many more details which are beyond the scope of this book and for which we refer the reader to the in-depth literature. But unfortunately – or thank goodness? – this subject is like an apple: we may have studied a 500-page treatise on it in every detail and yet do not know what it tastes like until we have bitten into it. But then at least three-quarters of the treatise is superfluous because of our own experience. For this reason, we recommend everyone to try it out for themselves. We should consider it worth spending half an hour twice a day to devote ourselves to the unknown side of life, when we have the remaining 23 hours at our unrestricted disposable for the other important or futile things. And we have seen in Elli's example that even when there are initial reservations the subjectively perceived benefit is so great that we are happy to take this little timeout for ourselves with pleasant anticipation and fulfilment. So why not have a holiday twice a day and go on a safari into the unknown but enticing land of our consciousness? In doing so, we do not have to fear a loss but rather a huge gain. For we saw in the previous chapter that we stopped learning and developing further because we were lacking impulses. But in the depths of our consciousness, where our individual consciousness encounters the collective and even the matrix of creation, there are impulses of an infinite number and variety. From there a subtle inkling rises up in us now and again in rare moments, whispering to us like a distant memory that there is another reality than that we are currently living.

Because of this memory we are also here now – in search of true health and the development towards our life purpose. Let's look into it, gather more concrete information, let it become knowledge and live this knowledge. In this way, our own experience will irrevocably turn this inkling into reality, into the foundation for a new future.

7. Is information everything?

"Any more questions, please?"

Samuk Deda let his searching gaze sweep over the crowded lecture room. He had just given a one-hour presentation on AyurVeda Ritam with the focus on "Diet" and was now offering the possibility of asking him direct questions.

A young man in the third row raised his hand and began to speak, after Samuk had gestured him to do so:

"I have been a vegetarian for almost two years, I mean a proper vegetarian, as you explained before, without meat, fish, eggs, mushrooms and algae – and I feel very well, in every respect. I must say that everything you talked about this evening is absolutely correct. I can only confirm it. But I have one problem and would like to have your advice about it: every day on my way home from work, I go past a stand selling sausages and it smells so tempting. I really have to restrain myself from becoming weak. But I know what harm such a sausage does in my body and so I always quickly walk past it."

The people in the room laughed.

"All the same I'm afraid," he went on, "that some time or other I will just not manage to restrain myself anymore. Can you give me some advice?"

"Yes, of course," replied Samuk, "bite into a sausage and enjoy it!"

"I beg your pardon?" the young man responded dumbfounded, "You mean …?

"Yes, buy one and bite into it! And next week tell us about your experience."

The young man was visibly surprised. He had certainly not expected this answer.

A week later, he attended the presentation with the focus on "Muskoskeletal and locomotor systems" and reported at the end:

"Well, you told me last week to report on my experience. The day after the presentation I actually went to the sausage stand and bought a sausage. I had a really bad conscience but you had expressly told me to do it. It smelt really delicious and I bit into it with great enjoyment. But then something strange happened: already as I was biting into it,

I felt the heavy fat spreading around my mouth and, in general, the sausage tasted quite different from what I knew from the past. When I swallowed the mouthful, I could really feel it blocking everything in my stomach. I felt quite strange and had no wish to bite into it again. So I just threw the rest in the rubbish bin. I then noticed the problem my digestion was having with the sausage and I was really glad when it finally had been expelled. This odour naturally reminded me of the past as well."

"And what happens now when you go past the sausage stand?" Samuk asked.

"You will laugh, but I don't go past it anymore. In the days afterwards I felt so sick only when I had the smell in my nose that I have made a big detour since then."

"You see," said Samuk, turning to the audience, "that's what happens when information becomes knowledge. I, in fact, told you that a proper diet has nothing to do with denial or prohibitions but only with proper consciousness. And our friend here will certainly never need a prohibition or any coercion again to be able to do without his sausage."

What had happened here? And what did the sentence with knowledge and information mean?

Let's first of all go into information in more detail, thereby considering the usual ways in which information is transmitted, such as language, radio, television, telephone, newspapers, books and others. From this we see that information does not really become information unless there is a receiver to take it in and understand it. Although radio, television and mobile radio waves of all types and frequencies buzz around our heads continually, we cannot, however, even perceive them without radios, television sets or cell phones. And to receive information, the devices also have to be tuned to the correct frequency or a mobile phone must have a telephone card with the correct number. But if the information is transmitted in a language we do not understand, it is not information for us either. That is why a book in Chinese is of just as little value to most Germans as a book in Arabic or a book without any print. So information does not seem to be something objective but depends to a high degree on the receiver and their readiness to receive.

An additional factor is that although information is mostly transmitted with the help of physical or chemical principles, it itself lies beyond matter and energy. Thus, for instance, an audiotape of Beethoven's ninth symphony cannot be distinguished from one of random noise by chemical or physical methodes of measurement. In quantitative terms, the two tapes are identical, although with the proper receiver the recorded tape can convey its information simultaneously to many thousands of people, for instance over the stereo facilities in a football stadium. Thus, quantity plays no part for the information. In this way, a whispered "yes" contains exactly the same information as one shouted across the countryside through a megaphone. What, in contrast, plays a considerable part is the syntax, i.e. the order and connection of the single elements. The words "spare", "pears" and "reaps" are made up of the same components, but due to their different sequence they contain different information. Even with identical syntax, different information may still result for different receivers. For instance, the word "gift" means a substance harmful to health for a German but a present for an English person.

So for any kind of information a receiver is needed who can enter into resonance with the transmitter of the information in such a way as was planned by the sender of the information. If the receiver possesses the correct code to be able to understand the information received correctly, the transmission of the information was successful. By no means do these processes necessarily have to take place via language. If, for example, someone nudges another person in a particular way and the latter notices and understands it, this is also transmission of information. Even physical methods of transmission are not, however, necessary at all costs, as in the case where two people who are close directly exchange emotions. At any rate, it is important to note that transmission of information is a very complex and subtle process, which, although it can utilise physical principles, has a content going far beyond matter and energy.

In our modern society, the flow of information has today assumed huge dimensions, but even this is negligible compared with our body. In the example of the family's drive to the countryside, we saw how many tasks our mind performs simultaneously. Every one of these is, in turn, based on countless single processes in an immeasurable number of individual cells, which all have to coordinate perfectly with each other. This requires precise transmission of information, which takes place in our body via the nerve cells by means of electric impulses and chemical neurotransmitters or via the bloodstream by means of messengers, i.e. hormones. These hormones are produced by the endocrine glands and then the blood takes them to the cells, which possess specific receptors in their cell walls that fit them like a key in a lock, thus triggering the desired reaction in the cell. These reactions might be an increase or a decrease in the production or further hormones or other substances. For example, when our driver realised that he had noticed the oncoming car on the other side much too late, he probably got an enormous shock. At that moment, his adrenal glands released an increased dose of adrenalin, signalling to his heart via the sympathetic system that it should beat faster and pump more blood, to his blood vessels that they should contract so as to increase blood pressure, to his liver that it should mobilise its glycogen reserves and release more glucose into the blood, to his gut that it should reduce digestion so that the energy required for it was available to the rest of the body, to his eyes that they should expand their pupils, and to his whole body that it should increase its basal energy rate and release more free fatty acids into the blood. All these processes take place in split seconds and are controlled by the brain. But as soon as he realised the danger was over and that he had been lucky, his body produced hormones inhibiting the sympathetic system again, thus restoring the body's normal state.

To give us a concrete idea of what a gigantic logistics and communication network our body actually is, let's simply convert it to everyday dimensions familiar to us. So let's imagine our body is a country inhabited by cells that are on average as large as humans. On this scale, our body would be some 120 km long. We thus have a "country" somewhat smaller than Germany but, nevertheless, with a population of 50 trillion inhabitants. They are all supplied centrally with food, and the waste disposal is also organised centrally. For that purpose, there is a transport system of some 7 billion km in length, on which 30 trillion energy transporters – the red corpuscles – are constantly moving. They supply each inhabitant individually and, in doing so, each one covers the entire network 2500 times a day on average. In comparison to this, Germany's road network is only 650,000 km long with some 50,000 km of railway tracks in addition and 50 million vehicles.

Furthermore, electrochemical telegraph cables criss-cross our "country": these are our nerve tracts, through which messages to the headquarters are sent at an equivalent speed of 150 – 3500 km per second and commands from the headquarters even at 8500 km per second. Moreover, many trillions of couriers are also travelling on the roads in this country: these are the hormones bringing individual information to particular inhabitants, not forgetting the 30 billion security officers, with even more than the same number on standby duty in the barracks. Alone this security system is a miracle in itself and would completely dwarf any Orwellian police state, which is, however, also indispensable in view of the cunning and dangerousness of possible opponents. And as the country's government is not only intelligent but wise as well, being and acting in harmony with the natural laws and striving for the well-being of all its subjects in harmony with the whole, no abuse of governmental authority is to be feared.

However, there is no kind of individual freedom in this country, for such free will is reserved to the human being alone in nature. And this human being has obviously had nothing better to do for generations than use their free will to destructive ends. This means that today the government of most "cell nations" has moved away from its course in line with natural law and has become a fatal danger for the entire national structure. For the government itself has begun to introduce noxious elements into the country and will not let itself be dissuaded from this despite the clearest of warnings from all sides. Besides, other modes of behaviour and ever worsening coordination and control bring numerous systems into disorder. Due to this schizophrenic situation the security forces become so confused that they either leave harmful elements in peace or attack harmless individuals, which manifests itself in the form of allergic reactions.

But let's return from these "political" considerations of "state policy" to the actual dimension of our body. We have seen that the mind's activity corresponds to an absolutely infinite number of chemical reactions taking place in many different parts of the body. And, in fact, every cell has its own power plant and hence its own metabolism and all mechanisms related to its function. For this purpose, it possesses a huge pool of information in its genes, although it only actually uses a tiny part of this. And the whole thing takes place in such close coordination and compliance with all other parts of the body that the comparison with the logistics and communications of a modern state is just too inept. Instead, we should rather think of a gigantic orchestra, in which 50 trillion musicians – could – play the symphony of true health in perfect harmony if they were not being continually obstructed and directly sabotaged by the conductor.

We do, in fact, always come back to the same point. For all re-search, all findings and all experiences with the human body show that its basic structures are so perfectly constructed and coordinated with each other that a perfect symphony in faultless harmony would be possible without any problem if wrong impulses did not continually cause confusion and disorder. These disruptions by no means always take place on the gross, material level. Rather, it is mostly "only" a question of information, which – as we have just seen – we cannot, however, get hold of physically or chemically. Yet, everyone can cer-tainly now easily imagine that the vast number of different processes and mechanisms means that innumerable possibilities for wrong influ-ences exist. Far more factors than we can consciously perceive with our brain constitute important information for our body. For instance, the body's surface is equipped with countless temperature sensors, which constantly measure the external temperature of every part of the body and regulate blood circulation and sweating accordingly so that inside the body the ideal temperature always prevails for the inner organs. The feet also play an important part in regulating the temper-ature, as they naturally give the ground temperature, which can differ distinctly from the air temperature. But if we wrap them up almost the whole time in shoes and socks, which impede or even completely stop the natural exchange of sweat and warmth, the body's entire heat balance can be disrupted. For this reason, experience has shown that when you have cold feet, it is often better to remove your shoes and socks altogether than to put an extra layer on top. In general, the temperature of the feet should be regulated primarily by movement and not so much by footwear, as it is of great importance for the whole body.

Other important information may be provided by colours, which often give indications of the state of foods, influence our emotional world or have even more far-reaching significance for our body. Thus, for instance, the colour of light indicates the time of day. Although this mostly happens unconsciously, our body still reacts to it unerr-ingly. Green and blue short-wave light of greater intensity, such as naturally prevails in the daytime, has an influence on the pineal gland or epiphysis. This endocrine gland, also often called the third eye, is directly connected to the retina of the eyes and from there receives information about where we are currently in our daily routine from the colour and intensity of the light. Incidentally, this also applies to most blind people as other nerves than the sight nerves are responsible for it. If no light or only weak or long-wave light reaches the eye, the epiphysis produces the hormone melatonin, which makes us sleepy, reduces our energy, prolongs our reaction time, thus preparing the body for sleep. If, on the other hand, bright, short-wave light shines into the eyes, the pineal gland stops producing melatonin, with the result that we wake up and stay awake. This mechanism explains why people in northern latitudes feel as if they are about to go to sleep during the long, dark and dreary winter months – which, in the long run, results in depression in some cases.

But the epiphysis not only produces melatonin but also some neurotransmitters and, in general, is of great importance for our entire hormonal balance. This means that light is not only for seeing but, at the same time, also influences our whole body. This influence, however, depends decisively on the type of light – hence on the information it contains – and the best, most natural light is provided by sunlight that reaches us unfiltered and unobstructed. Even the lenses of glasses change this information in such crucial areas that the body loses important impulses. This was noticed by Dr. John Ott, the father of full-spectrum light, as early as the 1960's when his glasses broke one day. At that time he was in a poor physical condition, he had arthritis in his hip and had to walk with a stick. An operation appeared to be unavoidable. Besides, he was very susceptible to infections. As he had heard how good sun is in such cases, he had a beach holiday in Florida, which did not, however, bring about any improvement. Back home, the mishap occurred with his glasses. And to his surprise, he promptly noticed a distinct improvement in his state of health within the following few days. He was even able to walk without a stick again. Since, as a photographer and producer of memo-motion films, he had already many years before noticed and investigated the effect of light of various spectra on the growth and development of plants and animals and had, above all, been struck by the negative impact of glass, which filters out UV rays, he soon began to suspect that his glasses might have something to do with the improvement in his health. Then he immediately booked another short holiday in Florida, which he this time spent very strictly without glasses or sunglasses. And he did indeed feel a noticeable improvement in his state after that holiday. The next time he had his hip examined the result was really surprising and there was no more talk of the hip operation already planned.

Dr. Ott subsequently did numerous investigations into the impact of light of differing wave-lengths and also published several books on this topic. Thus, it has indisputably been proved today that natural sunlight with its full spectrum is an important and essential part of our "diet." Even though the mechanisms have not all yet been fully clarified, the experiments do show unequivocally that regular and sufficient solar irradiation has a positive impact on general health, the immune system, circulation, blood test results, cholesterol level, calcium metabolism, fitness and stamina, mental well-being, social behaviour, potency and fertility and brings about decisive improvements in diseases such as diabetes, cancer, arteriosclerosis of the brain or hyper-activity in children. In this, it cannot be ruled out that the impact of solar irradiation occurs for the most part directly on the blood. For the haem of the red blood colouring only differs essentially from chlorophyll, which carries out photosynthesis in plants, in that the former contains an iron ion and the latter a magnesium ion.

Dr. Ott showed in an experiment with mimosas that there are many other not understood factors and correlations. These sensitive plants have their stems directed upwards and their leaves opened during the day and fold their leaves and bend their stems downwards at sunset. They remain in this position until sunrise, when they unfold again. Dr. Ott first found out that the mimosas also maintain this behaviour unchanged in dark rooms with complete exclusion of sunlight, so that it appeared that they possess a sort of memory for the daily schedule. But then he placed some plants in a coalmine 200m underground and the plants immediately adopted their night position until they were brought above ground again. The artificial lighting in the mine did not seem to have any significance for them.

This observation makes it clear that the mimosas react to different information from the sun than simply light. That is certainly also the case with humans, even though no scientific investigations have yet been done concerning this. The special position of the pineal gland at the base of the brain at any rate leaves room for speculation in this direction. At the same time, evidence has recently been mounting that the pineal gland also reacts to electromagnetic radiation from power lines, computer monitors or mobile telephone systems, namely negatively for the body's hormonal balance and its functioning on the cellular level. The possible consequences range from miscarriages to birth defects, neural impairments, circulatory problems, hyperactivity and even cancer and leukaemia. Dr. Ott also played a pioneering role here, when, as early as the 1980's, he published an experiment in which he placed a blood sample directly in front of a switched-on monitor. Thereupon, so-called rouleaux formations, i.e. clusters of red corpuscles in the shape of rolls of coins, formed in the blood within five minutes. When he then exposed the same blood sample to weak UV light instead, the structure of the blood became normal again within five minutes.

In general, we see from these examples what an enormous amount of information our body is continually receiving, mostly without us being aware of it. Much of this is necessary for its smooth functioning, but much of it also has a disruptive or even harmful impact. If we realise alone on account of the last experiment what a diversity of radiation sources – electric power lines, electric sockets, electric devices, television and computer screens, remote controls, cordless telephones or mobile phones – we are constantly exposed to, it should become absolutely clear to us that this cannot remain without influence on our body or mind. For even if scientists are still arguing about the influences, threshold levels, ceilings, impact mechanisms, etc., a huge amount of information that is certainly not in harmony with natural bodily functions is at any rate continually being transmitted to our body. And if, in this connection, we even think back to Professor Grinberg's experiments on the influence of a meditating person's brainwaves, which are not even physically measurable outside the body in terms of their field strength, here we also ought to ask ourselves the serious question as to what we want and are striving for – the development towards true health or the doubtful benefits of a permanent stream of information and constant availability. The information which we constantly allow to wash over us mostly unfiltered from the media, often has no direct relevance whatsoever for our life. Yet, we absorb it and let it work in us, whereby each of us can count on three fingers what harm scenes of violence, crime, atrocities, injustice, etc. do to us. We know from experience that every glance, every gesture, every word and even wordless silence actually contain a treasury of information for our mind and our emotions, even if we are not directly conscious of it. Thus, we can often see how someone feels from looking at their face or hear what someone really wants to express from the mere tone of their voice. Likewise, a good or bad mood is automatically contagious, even when no concrete initiatives are taken in this respect. What harm we are doing to ourselves when we let in all kinds of information, which has not even been selected by ourselves but by some editor or other according to doubtful criteria! A headline is mostly only considered interesting if it is clearly negative. Positive news is hardly ever to be heard for this reason, although even today a lot of positive and gratifying things are happening in the world. Of course, it is important to be informed about certain fundamental things, but a weekly summary on Sunday would suffice for this as, in addition, it would no longer contain all the news which was already out of date the following day. Wouldn't it be appropriate to think seriously about what important fundamental information, for which it is worth being constantly up-to-date, really is?

For our body as well, contact with any form of matter or energy is connected to information which triggers specific reactions in our organism. We have already seen how every step with bare feet triggers a whole stream of reflex impulses to the entire body, which similarly applies to any contact with the skin as well. The skin, in turn, likewise reacts to influences of light of the most diverse kinds and to substances that affect it via the air, water or clothing. We receive particularly intensive information via smells and tastes. Our tongue alone has more than 9000 taste cells, each of which sends its messages to the brain and thus to the rest of the body.

If we take all of this into consideration, we can understand that a walk over a meadow in the summer, only with the socially necessary minimum of clothing, provokes a true fortissimo for the symphony of the orchestra represented by our body. Our skin and our hair rejoice at each caressing touch of the wind, which, carries a multiplicity of delicious fragrances with it as well as oxygen. The sun shining from an intensively blue sky, fractured in countless shades of green in the grasses and leaves and also in the myriads of dabs of colour in the great diversity of flowers in all nuances of the colour spectrum, pervades our whole body, not only our eyes but also our skin, giving precious comforting warmth to our innermost being. Our ears take in the concert of twittering birds and the humming and buzzing insects, filling the air against the mighty background of the rustling of the trees in the rhythm of the wind to the playful accompaniment of the gurgling of a little stream. These basic instruments are varied with numerous capricious and grounding, invigorating or calming sub-parts, creating a holistic impact on body, mind and soul which continues long after the end of the walk.

But likewise we can also well understand how much disharmony and cacophony occur in the symphony when we spend time in a modern factory or office building during our normal daily life. During this time our skin is mostly rubbed or sprayed with sticky, pore-blocking chemical substances, whose toxic solvents penetrate the body, triggering immune reactions. Their odours mix with all kinds of undefinable synthetic smells from the environment and the used, stale air to produce an absolutely breath-taking cocktail, which our nose would prefer to block out, as it brings devastating consequences for our respiratory tract and lungs. At the same time, our skin is enveloped in synthetic fibres, which disrupt its electrostatic exchange and the regulation of its temperature and moisture, even leading to irritation due to the substances they contain. Our eyes have to use all their strength to be able to fulfil their tasks in the unnatural, flickering light and our ears are confused by a jumble of strange, loud and soft noises of the oddest frequencies. On top of this, the numerous important sub-parts are lacking, screened off by the Faraday cage of a steel concrete building and by hermetically sealed energy-saving windows. Instead, other disruptions of harmony are created by the building fabric and the building materials, by the one-sided, unnatural movement and posture and by the fundamental hecticness. With such a cast, the perfect masterwork of true health cannot, at any rate, be realised even with the best of conductors. There you can save yourself any rehearsing from the start.

The greatest flow of information in our body undoubtedly takes place through our mouth. We have already seen how well our tongue alone is equipped for assessing taste and we can indeed perceive so many different nuances of taste that we lack the vocabulary for most of them. Yet, taste is only a small part of the infinitely multi-layered information that passes through our mouth. We see that most clearly in medicine or drugs, where just a few drops suffice to bring about enormous and sometimes dramatic effects in the body. These can partially be comprehended biochemically, but their complexity mostly goes far beyond current scientific understanding. That is particularly clear with homeopathic remedies, which for a long time were dismissed by quantitative science as humbug, having only an imagined effect. And it is indeed so that particularly the highly potentised remedies only contain a few or no molecules at all of the active component in their solvent in arithmetic terms, because of the degree to which they have been diluted. So how are they to have any effect? In contrast, there have, nevertheless, been numerous unequivocal reports on the success of homeopathic treatments since the foundation of homeopathy by Samuel Hahnemann in 1796. Thus, its effectiveness is undeniable. As in so many other areas, the key here lies in the information. We have already seen that information lies beyond physics and chemistry, even if it utilises related natural laws. The complicated and time-consuming process of producing homeopathic high potencies seems to have succeeded in transmitting the information of the effective component to the carrier substance, even to an increasing extent the more they are diluted.

Such effects are easily comprehensible with water, as, on account of the spatial arrangement of their components and their charge distribution, the water molecules spontaneously tend to assemble in larger units called clusters. We indirectly recognise this from the astonishing fact that after ice has melted, water reduces its volume when the temperature goes on rising and does not start to expand until the temperature is above 4°C. This anomaly shows that large-scale structures still exist in water in its liquid state and break up below 4° C, allowing a more compact, space-saving distribution of the molecules with an initially decreasing volume. But such clusters still exist at higher temperatures, only with the normal thermic dilation predominating because of the increased movement of the molecules. Due to this property, more than any other substance, water has the capacity to store information. For a receiver who can get into resonance with it, any cluster configuration signifies specific information, even if – as with the tape of Beethoven's ninth – nothing is physically measurable.

Without knowing about these mechanisms, Hahnemann succeeded in developing a process enabling him to transfer the information of the active components he had used as a base to the solvent – mostly alcohol or cane sugar in this case. The effect of a highly potentised homeopathic remedy thus does not depend on the substances it contains but on the information contained in it. This very fact makes homeopathy into a stomping ground for self-medication for many people, since they think it cannot actually do harm and there are no side-effects either. But what a huge impact pure information can have in a particular context can be seen from the seemingly inconsequential message "Y-3, Q-3, B-2, C-1", which Paul Tibbets, the pilot of the B-29 bomber Enola Gay, received on 6 August 1945 at 7.30 am local time. For him it meant that the weather conditions were good above the Japanese city of Hiroshima, to which he thereupon steered his bomber and then dropped the world's first atomic bomb at 8.15 am. We must not underestimate the significance and potential impact of information. For the very reason that homeopathic remedies do not have an effect on the material level but on the informational level, they are less straightforward than allopathic medicines. They can thus have a direct influence on the mind and emotions and there provoke worse side-effects than directly physiological ones. Therefore the greatest care should also be taken here, and we should, if possible, rely on the pure and unadulterated substances and information nature provides our body with.

Hippocrates was undoubtedly more correct when he uttered the principle as long as 2,000 years ago: "Let food be thy medicine and medicine be thy food." This expresses a basic trust that God's nature provides everything we need for our health at the right time, in the right amount and in the right combination. And, in fact, pharmaceutical medicine has done nothing else in essence to date but isolate effective components from plants or make synthetic imitations of them. However, it does not seem to be aware that it will never be able to come close to the effectiveness of nature. For although it may succeed in imitating the substances, it will never artificially obtain the correct informational content. It is indeed so that any alteration or processing simultaneously involves a change in the information contained – and never a positive one. For as we have seen, with information – unlike with pure matter – not only the components it contains are important but their arrangement and syntax are also crucial. In this respect, however, those responsible lack the necessary overview of the correlations, apart from being completely unconscious that they have to do with a complex informational structure in this case. It is as if someone gets a hexadecimally coded computer program but only sees it as a long text consisting of the characters 0 – 9 and A – F. If they at some point find the word "FACE" in it, they then think that the text has something to do with a face and the lines before and after it contain some useful information on this topic. If they then "isolate" these lines, they destroy the whole program – naturally without knowing it – and do not have anything in their hands even coming close to what they think they have found.

Although this explanation will certainly make sense to most people, almost all of us still make these very mistakes, namely in preparing their food. Instead of taking food and eating it as nature has provided it, we process it. We isolate, mix, freeze, heat, refine, season, etc. and are not in the slightest aware of what we are actually wreaking. In addition, there is everything that we do not do ourselves but is manipulated by the food industry mostly without our knowledge to preserve food, to make it easy to spread, meltable or free-flowing, to liquefy or solidify it, to make it blendable, airy, loose, coloured, sticky, crunchy, crisp, firm, etc. or to prevent it forming lumps or flakes, drying out, hardening or suchlike. Today we actually no longer eat real food but well-packed, effectively marketed chemical cocktails, which with the use of tricks create the illusion of traditional, natural, good, solid food. "Like grandmother's food, fresh from the garden!" But every clearly thinking person must wonder at least once where pieces of "real" vegetables, potatoes or meat suddenly come from in the package soup, which was pure powder two minutes before. It is equally surprising that the instant roast also browns in the microwave although no grilling process takes place there.

Earlier in the book, we spoke in detail about food, although mainly about its material aspect. The related transmission of information was only mentioned in connection with Martha and her depression. However, it is an absolutely crucial factor everywhere. For just as an animal trembles in panic for fear of death with every fibre of its being and every cell of its body shortly before being slaughtered, its meat – in whatsoever form – later represents coded fear, aggression and despair, and that is the information everyone absorbs into their body and consciousness when they eat meat. It makes no great difference whether the meat originates from happy cows on the meadow or in a factory farm. For the moment of death is of the same quality in both cases – for the "happy" animal even with the additional smack of perfidious underhandedness, while the animal from industrial farming is rather put out of its misery.

In this case, the mechanisms are to some extent easy to understand but, nevertheless, only relatively few people think about them. So what about all the small but important elements of information which are otherwise dispensed to us in food, without our suspecting anything and without being able to follow what harm they do in the symphony of our body! Quantity plays no part in this, as we have already seen, for a whispered "No" is still a "No". But our body receives all this information in an unerring way and also reacts accordingly. Rudolph

Virchow, father of modern pathology, made a remarkable discovery in this respect in 1897. He was the first to realise that diseases had something to do with the body's cells and that the crucial stages from break-out to healing play out on this level. In connection with his investigations related to this, he found that the number of white blood cells always distinctly increased a short time after eating. This phenomenon, also known as "digestive leucocytosis" still today, presented a puzzle. For normally leucocytosis, i.e. an increase in the number of white blood cells, means that the body is fighting intruders. The leucocytes, in fact, constitute a main part of our immune defence system and have the task of detecting substances or cells which are dangerous for the body – also those produced by the body itself, like cancer cells – of marking them, rendering them harmless or simply devouring them. Although nobody was able to explain this digestive leucocytosis, because the findings were unequivocal and easily reproducible it was accepted and established as a physiological phenomenon – until the Swiss doctor Kouchakoff from Lausanne had another look at the issue in the 1920's. He carried out several hundred experiments, the results of which were published in 1930 in Paris at the first international microbiology congress and presented in an extended and more detailed form in a publication of the Société vaudoise des sciences naturelles in Lausanne. In it, he stated that digestive leucocytosis is not a physiological but a pathological phenomenon. His investigations had, in fact, revealed that it does not occur if one eats uncooked food, with his even indicating in his second publication a so-called critical temperature of various foods as a maximal temperature for heating them. This temperature, however, lies consistently below 100°C. Furthermore, he found that the incidence of leucocytosis is lower or absent if one eats at least 10% of each food raw at every meal.

On the basis of these findings, we can establish that our body has problems with how we process our food before eating. In this respect, today's problematic additives in industrial foods certainly did not yet play any part in Kouchakoff's experiments, as they did not exist then. Temperature was the crucial thing according to his findings. And that is not astonishing, as we can comprehend today with our much greater nutritional, physiological knowledge. Indeed, we now know that if food is heated to above 48°C, it begins to change chemically: proteins coagulate, carbohydrates caramelise, fatty acids alter their structure, up to half the vitamins are destroyed, minerals are converted back to their anorganic form, which is useless to the body, fibrous substances break up so that they lose their function, which is so important for the gut, and the enzymes are completely destroyed. The denaturing of protein already starts at 42°C, which is the reason that fever becomes life-threatening when it reaches this temperature.

Here, it is crucial to understand that the macromolecules which build up our body and exercise important functions in it are so complex and specialised that not only the composition and arrangement of their parts is important, but also their spatial structure. Thus, for instance, there are two forms of lactic acid, which are as similar to each other just as two hands are. That means that they consist of exactly the same parts in the same arrangement, but differ inversely like a mirror image. And this small spatial difference is actually noticeable in a decisive manner. For the body only produces the so-called clockwise L(+) form and can also easily digest this. In contrast, the anticlockwise D(−) form normally does not exist in the body at all and can also only be metabolised in food indirectly. Here we are thus confronted with a subtle informational element, which nevertheless plays a big part for the body. Another example is prions, which are responsible for mad cow disease and Creutzfeldt-Jakob disease. These are, in fact, actually the body's own protein molecules, which, however, display a different spatial convolution and are thus harmful. These examples show that the spatial structure of macromolecules is anything but secondary. And this is the very thing that changes first when they are heated, with the molecules losing their biological effectiveness and even possibly becoming harmful if the body still uses them. The unsaturated fatty acids in high-quality vegetable oils, for instance, lose their curved structure and become straight. This means that they behave like saturated fatty acids and likewise start to clot and form deposits in the artery walls. If they are built into the wall of a cell in the body in this form, they naturally cannot fulfil the expected function and cause considerable disruptions in the whole cell metabolism. Enzymes also lose their spatial structure above 42°C and, thus, their biological function, which consists in facilitating chemical reactions in the body or even making them possible at all. For this, the digestive system produces a whole range of specific digestive enzymes, and every cell requires such molecules for its correct functioning. To date, 5000 different enzymes have been discovered. It is estimated, however, that up to 100,000 are necessary to maintain all bodily functions. Plant foods, particularly fruits, but also other parts of plants, to a smaller extent, by nature contain a large quantity of enzymes, which the plant needs for its own metabolism. They are, for example, responsible for the ripening of the fruit and also for it becoming over-ripe in the course of time. These phyto-enzymes can be a valuable aid to our digestive system, as they virtually perform the same digestive processes as take place in our stomach and gut. For this reason, typical herbivores in the animal kingdom have – as we saw in chapter 4 – a structured stomach, which allows the enzymes contained in food to continue with their pre-digestion before the body's digestive juices come into full play. Besides, it has also even been found in radioactive marking experiments that an astonishingly large part of the enzymes in food pass through the stomach undamaged, continue to perform their function in the small intestine and even enter the body's cells in the blood to continue working there. All that makes it clear what a great value enzymes in food have – provided they are not destroyed by heat, which already happens at temperatures above 42°C. The body has to expend much more energy for the digestion of cooked food, as it, firstly, has to produce all the required enzymes itself and, secondly, only manages with the greatest effort, or even not at all, to break down the coagulated protein and the caramelised carbohydrates into their single components.

Heating has a negative impact even on minerals, although they themselves are not sensitive to heat. They are, in fact, hard for the body to make use of in their elementary form and should therefore be embedded in a molecule complex made of organic molecules. But if this complex is destroyed, the atoms or ions of the mineral substances revert to an anorganic form, in which the body can utilise them as little as it could a rusty nail or a piece of copper wire.

With this understanding, it is no longer astonishing that the body reacts to cooked food in the same way as if it was having to defend itself against harmful foreign bodies. That is indeed what it is having to do! For the use of heat has so altered the natural nutrients that the body hardly recognises them and can only use them with a great effort, if at all. Not for nothing is the pancreas, which has to produce most of these enzymes, twice as large in a modern human being than in a herbivorous animal in relation to body weight. And experiments with rats have shown that their pancreases gain about a quarter of their weight within six months when they are fed only cooked food not containing any enzymes of its own.

Here, we indeed have to do with a very subtle problem, about which even a diet-conscious person will not find any information in the list of ingredients in their food. Neither is it primarily a material problem, for most of the components are still present as such – but simply in a slightly altered form. Yet, this altered form entails such a drastic change in the transmission of information that the situation is completely upside down for the body. In this respect, we have said nothing at all about additives, which we are fobbed off with – legally or illegally – in foods today. Particularly in recent times, the food industry has discovered enzymes as wonder helpers – which do not have to be stated on the packaging –, which, for instance, improve the flavour of tinned peas, generate the mild taste of instant coffee, increase the yield in the production of fruit juices and also of cold-pressed olive oil or make marmalade, noodles and crackers last longer. The enzymes used for this - even in plant foods - are partially of animal origin, for example hen's eggs. What a mumbo-jumbo of information for our body! For the enzymes also go on working in our body unceasingly. And so far nobody knows – or is interested in – what harm they do. But, anyway, we must not be under any illusions. For even if all ingredients had to be completely listed, that would only increase transparency of the substances but not of their information. Thus, it is, for example, customary to produce the flavour of strawberries or raspberries and also of vanilla from wood shavings. Such flavours may even be described as natural, since wood is, after all, a natural basic material. Incidentally, that also makes it understandable how the food scandals much published in the media, in which toxic residue from wood preservative were found in fruit yoghurts, were able to come about. But all kinds of industrial waste are used in the production of our food to reduce costs. Thus, the "valuable" iodine used to artificially enrich more and more foods often originates from production residues of the chemical industry, the ballast added to bread from the residues from breweries or margarine factories and the gelatine in yoghurt from slaughterhouse waste. Furthermore, emulsifiers for many – also "pure vegetable" – foods are made from the fat of slaughtered animals and additives for chocolate or biscuits from pig's blood. In addition to all this, there is a no longer manageable list of synthetic additives, from which an information cocktail of the worst kind is concocted, which is to blame for the most conflicting unknown and unexpected reactions in our body, but also in our mind and soul. In this respect, the exclusively applicable principle of profit maximisation has even already gone so far that a Japanese scientist has developed a process for making a raw material for instant meals from sewage sludge.

This may certainly lead to disgusted protest from many people, but a closer look shows that through our drinking water we have for years been supplying our body with treated waste water from industrial plants or sewage plants, which is pumped out of the major rivers into our water pipes by the central long-distance water supply. Of course it is treated, cleaned and the substances it contains strictly controlled. But if we keep in mind the principle of potentiation discovered by Samuel Hahnemann in connection with homeopathy and water's "capacity for remembering" described above, the comparison of our tap water inevitably suggests itself with a highly potentised remedy, in which the original substance has been carefully diluted out but its information nevertheless remains, all the stronger and more effective. All chemical analyses, even with the most modern and sensitive apparatus, will not provide any further information here, since for them the treated Rhine water is of the same quality as fresh spring water from the Alps – and they may be right on the level of the substances contained. But with the same argument and on the basis of the same apparatus, we can also use the pure solvent instead of homeopathic remedies. If the high potencies do have a profound impact on the body, although they no longer contain anything of the original active components, then water – and with it all foods – also has an impact, going back to all the substances and treatment processes it has come in contact with. And then we should immediately think about this information, which we continually feed ourselves with. Nature – even inanimate, anorganic nature – obviously has a memory and transmits information which for analytical researchers is as inconceivable and impossible to measure as Beethoven's ninth on the tape. For they do not have a receiver for it and only examine the material properties of the tape. Yet, our body is a highly sensitive receiver and our present state shows that it receives data which destroy it.

It is, of course, correct that we have less and less influence on the air we breathe, the water we drink and even the food we eat, but we also have to be aware that we are all part of the society and system which has let things get that far. If we really care about our health and our development, we have to make decisions and start taking control of our lives again. And the more people do that, the sooner the harmful and pathological aberrations will cease. Fortunately it is easy for us.

For we do not need to develop a complicated method to supply our body with the proper nutrients and the correct information. Rather we only need to leave the basics to nature and its mechanisms again. There, everything has, in fact, been working since the beginning of creation in such perfect fine tuning that the optimal requirements for us also issue from it. Thus, there is no better information system for the air than the swaying tops of trees and bushes with their swinging leaves, no more perfect information system for water than the layers of rocks and minerals in the soil and no more perfect information system for our nutrition than plants, each of which with its grandiose intelligence in perfect attunement with the seasons, temperature, moisture and the entire ecosystem produces from the sun's energy and the minerals in the soil a unique composition of nutrients, trace elements, flavours, enzymes and information, which could not be more ideal for our body.

Let's get away from the erroneous idea that we can do better than the infinite intelligence which produced us including our intelligence, and not only that but all the other parts of animate and inanimate nature as well, in perfect coordination with one another. In every single ripe fruit and every seed, precious treasures are concealed which even all the world's chemical laboratories together could not produce in anything coming near to this diversity and perfection. As soon as we go and try to extract, isolate or concentrate them, valuable elements of their structure and composition are lost. Light, oxygen or heat alter the shape of the complex molecules, rendering them inferior or even worthless for our body. All the nutritional supplements in the world can never make up for this loss. But it is this loss which leaves us eternally dissatisfied, unfulfilled and unsatiated. Our body is hungry, although our stomach is already overfilled and our body is overweight. It is not hungering for the basic components of its existence, which is more than amply provided for, but for the information "between the lines", for those subtle messages in the form of molecules or molecular structures with a memory function, which convey the real essence of life to us and are necessary at all costs for existence to become life, functioning to become development, sound to become music and health to become true health.

Nevertheless, we should also pay great attention to when and in which form we let our body have information. For just as most of us protest about the unsolicited sending of post, faxes or emails, which has in recent times been much frowned upon as spam, our body also has to deal with every piece of information, whether it wanted it, needs it or not. But we practise such spamming or unrequested input of information with every "little bite" in between meals, with every kind of seasoning and with every little glass or cup of something, except pure water. Herbs and teas are also highly concentrated carriers of information and ought to be administered to the body with this awareness – when it needs them as medicine, or when it clearly wants them – not out of habit, boredom or on social occasions. Otherwise they will also cause disharmony.

At any rate, we should strictly avoid the destructive sounds of death, which unfortunately nowadays vibrate in most people at every second bite at the least. For they drown everything and stifle the entire symphony of life in the course of time. Likewise, everything that disrupts internal transmission and processing of information in our body is to be avoided. This primarily means alcohol, for it is known to impede neural processes, even killing nerve cells. Although there are still people who hold the opinion that alcohol is conducive to health in small quantities, this is opposed to all physiological findings and is probably only due to these people being in the thrall of alcohol themselves. Here as well, every individual has to decide of their own free will what is important to them. In this, it is however, crucial that it is clear to them that any glass of alcohol – be it ever so small – befogs the mind in its functions. Even when out of indifference due to habit we no longer directly perceive it, it still has its concrete impact somewhere, for example through an immune reaction being left out, a digestive step being incorrectly performed or a brick being faultily replaced during the renewal of our body, as described in chapter 3. The same mistakes may also be caused by other neurotoxins or drugs, stress or lack of sleep. We bear a large portion of responsibility in having such a complex system as our body at our disposal. But, at the same time, if correctly handled, it can – and will – enable us to achieve highs which completely dwarf any flight to the moon.

To conclude the discussion about nutrition, we now want to have a closer look at one class of foods which we have only mentioned marginally up to now, namely milk and dairy products. Milk is a problematic food, shrouded in a whole array of myths and strong emotional associations – probably from our own childhood. But first and foremost with all mammals it is the natural food for a new-born baby up to the moment when it itself can eat. For this the composition and informational content of milk are coordinated in an absolutely perfect manner and adjust themselves precisely to the baby's needs. So cow's milk is not intended for humans but for a cow's baby, which does not double its weight within six months like a human baby but within 1½ months and already weighs 150 kg after one year. That is why – as we saw in chapter 4 – it contains more than three times as much protein and more than four times as much calcium as a human mother's milk. For this very reason cow's milk is seen as the ideal food in times when more and more people are suffering from a calcium deficiency and many women get osteoporosis in old age. But, firstly, pasteurisation renders approximately half the calcium in milk useless to humans and, secondly, the body uses more calcium to deal with the high amounts of protein than milk supplies it with. In low-fat milk, this balance is even more negative, as it largely lacks the fat needed to absorb calcium. In addition, pasteurisation and, above all, ultra-heat treatment completely denature the valuable enzymes in milk. Besides that, their inner structure is also altered by homogenisation, in which the milk is pressed through fine nozzles under enormous pressure so that its fat is better distributed in small droplets. This process releases substances from the membranes of the fat droplets, which can lead to intolerance reactions.

According to our classification in chapter 4, milk and dairy products are not to be classed among animal products but among plant foods, as they are not attacked by putrefying bacteria but by lactic acid bacteria. From this point of view, there is therefore no objection to them in principle, which, however, does not apply to long-life milk and the other strongly altered dairy products offered on the market today. For only in the rarest of cases do these turn sour, but rather they putrefy or form mould and are therefore harmful for humans. Anyone who, after these considerations and those in chapter 4, still thinks they cannot or do not want to do without milk is therefore strictly advised to consume raw and, if possible, untreated milk from grass-fed cows. For anything else is strongly denatured and therefore harmful to health. Thus, milk intolerance is mostly less due to the milk itself than to the processing methods it is subjected to. An exception to this is the production of sour milk or natural yoghurt, as this does not denature milk but rather upgrades it. For the metabolic activity of the lactic acid bacteria vitalises it and makes it easier to digest.

Another extremely important factor in connection with dairy products is the amount. For as they are extremely highly concentrated foods, they should be consumed sporadically at the most and only in small quantities. This applies all the more for processed dairy products, as their concentration of nutrients is considerably greater. For example, roughly a tenfold amount of milk is required to produce cheese. Traditional small farmers, who were common in previous centuries and are still to be found in some parts of the world today, certainly came much nearer to these quantities than today's industrial mass production does. For, at that time, milk was only available as long as a cow had a calf and also only as much as the calf left over. In this way, milk was thus temporarily part of people's diet now and again or was preserved in the form of small amounts of cheese for the remaining time. But there was also nothing for long periods. Today's usual production and consumption amount, however, are an insanity, which not only costs our health dear but also means a brutal fate for cows. For this reason, the aftertaste and undertone of mistreatment and death unavoidably resonate today in every dairy product, which certainly does not contribute positively to our health and development.

In general, the fact is and simply remains that – regardless of processing and amount – cow's milk and the products made from it contain the information of becoming a cow, which they pass on. That is why, apart from any considerations of taste and physiology, it must, in turn, be clear to everyone what their goal is and what information they want to feed their body and mind with.

Now we have spoken a lot about information and also dealt with a lot of fundamental and important information in the previous chapters. But, as so often after reading an informative book or attending an interesting lecture, the question raises itself: "What now?" This question in itself already shows the limited value of pure information. For alone the ingesting of information from a book, a computer or a person with our mind has not changed anything about the information itself. It has only, so to speak, been copied on to an additional storage space, where it can go on waiting for something to happen to it, like the book or computer discs collecting dust on the shelf. However, we are more than just an information storage medium. For unlike books or computers, we have the possibility of implementing, using and living information. This means that we can make something disproportionately more valuable and more complex out of the information. We can transform it to another dimension to a certain extent. We can change it into knowledge.

The word "know" is unfortunately mostly a synonym for "being informed" in our language today, so that the transformation of information into knowledge we just mentioned does not look very special. But the knowledge we are talking about here is something quite different, which is why we would rather use the Sanskrit word "Veda" for it. An inkling of the difference between conventional so-called knowledge and genuine knowledge – Veda – can perhaps be gained if we compare the binary code of a programmed computer game, i.e. an absolutely infinite sequence of '0's' and '1's', with the program actually running with all its colour, sound and movement effects. Or even better, if the sequence of letters 'I LOVE YOU' is compared with the state of the person who receives this message from the right person in the right situation. Thus, knowledge goes far beyond intellect and embraces mind, body and soul to an equal extent. Not until we have grasped something intellectually, believe it emotionally and it has physically "become second nature" do we know it. However, it then fills every cell of our body, every corner of our soul and every sector of our mind. We become it and live it with every fibre of our consciousness. These may sound like very big words, but every couple who recently fell in love, every loving mother or every real artist knows what is meant. When a certain piece of information has become knowledge, there is no longer the slightest trace of doubt, reservation or protest. We then implement it spontaneously and correctly in every situation. For instance, if someone threatens us with a knife, we perhaps do not take it really seriously at first, even when the blade is at our throat. But once it is clear that the person with the knife really means it seriously, our mind, body and emotions react in an unequivocal way. If someone then rescues us from this life-threatening situation, no reflection or external impulse is necessary for us to be grateful to them. Rather, our entire world of emotions vibrates, every cell in our body quivers and our mind literally falls over itself in deeply felt, genuine gratitude.

The question that now arises – particularly in view of the many aspects discussed in this book – is: How do we turn this information into knowledge? That is the threshold everyone must cross when they want to change their diet, lose weight permanently, stop smoking or give up some other habits. Thus, we may intellectually possess all the information on what harm cigarette smoke does to the body or in emotional terms feel awfully unwell with our body's surplus pounds, but as long as the body does not go along with it and does not assimilate this information, we can make all the efforts in the world and will still not manage to get rid of our problems. Remember the young man with the sausage. He had had a completely vegetarian diet for two years and had had good experiences with it, as he himself confirmed. Nevertheless, the penny had not yet completely dropped in some corner of his consciousness. The smell of the sausages triggered in some cells of his body impulses from old, year-long habits, which one sector of his mind also remembered and which, at the same time, reawakened some long forgotten emotions. Thus, an appetite actually arose, which he was only able to control with strong will power, making him increasingly unfree in the long run. When he then, on Samuk Deda's advice, overrode his actually founded intellectual reservations – which was by no means easy for him, as he himself described –, the wonderful thing happened. All the cells in his body without exception had the concrete experience of what a physiological effect such a sausage has. In this way, he became conscious intellectually, emotionally and physically that this feeling of desire was not a need but only a distant memory, lacking any real foundation and totally inconsistent with his present state. This memory was deleted by his new current experience and overwritten by his new bodily feeling. In this way, he henceforth reacted with aversion on all levels, without his brain having to defy other areas of his consciousness. The information had become knowledge.

But had the young man not manipulated himself by pushing through a particular diet on an intellectual level, which simply had to inevitably lead to the scene described? Yes and no. Of course, he had used his intellect to change his deep-seated eating habits. But, in doing so, his physical experience during the entire time clearly showed that it was good and right for him. For, without the sausage stand on his way home, he would not have had any doubts, which would certainly not have been the case with a real negative manipulation. Secondly, the experience with the sausage would have had quite a different outcome if his mind had actually curtailed his body's elementary needs.

To transform information into real knowledge, it is, first of all, necessary to gain experience. For, without concrete personal experience, we do not get beyond the grey theory collecting dust in books. Information is not filled with life until it is implemented, and the resulting experience then shows whether the theory is correct or not. In the overwhelming majority of cases, it is the mind which initiates such a development. For nowadays information can be conveyed through the intellect in the simplest and most direct way. The soul generally has the least problems with changes in the direction of natural laws. For it is the part of us which is still most in harmony with creation. It is often even so that it would change certain things of itself, were it not impeded by the mind stuffed full of scientific information and the body spoilt by wrong habits. Although it also likes to hold on to pleasant feelings, such as the rustic atmosphere when roasting sausages by the campfire in a circle of close friends outdoors on a clear summer evening, or the comforting, homey feeling when eating hot chicken soup at the table with the family after a sledge ride in the snow. But here the important thing is not the food but, above all, the feelings, which emerge when grilling potatoes as well or eating a warm bean soup – provided the situation fits.

Our body has a more difficult time. Although it is the one that has to suffer most directly because of our wrong behaviour, it is also most spoilt by its one-sidedness and addictive features. That is why it is the most challenged by a change of diet as it has to alter its entire biochemistry. Paradoxically, this is made even harder for it by the mind of all things, since the latter mostly cannot let go of certain patterns of behaviour, thus repeatedly confronting the body with its old behaviour through the use of special memories or purposefully induced situations.

In general, we again see that knowledge is a holistic phenomenon. Pure information is just as inadequate in this respect as pure faith. Certainty, security and real life are only created through the interaction and the mutual reinforcement of body, mind and soul. Thus, it is important to apply body and mind in equal measure when transforming information into knowledge. The emotions then appear almost automatically from the resulting experience. In this process, the mind mainly needs the information and the motivation to implement it, at least experimentally at first. At the same time, it is important for it to let go and allow things to happen. The body, in contrast, first of all needs cleansing to free it from the addictive and irritating substances preventing it from returning to its innate functioning. And then it also needs information and experience to show it the way to new functional mechanisms. Those are the elements we talked about in the previous chapters: leaving out harmful and misinforming dietary components, adequate regular exercise and, above all, cultivation of hunger - the body's best and most natural cleansing mechanism -, and simultaneously the regular practice of Ritam Samation, which helps the mind let go, at the same time conveying valuable impulses to it from the matrix level.

All these measures are bundled into a harmonious and harmonising whole in Pancha Sama Ritam, the most intensive and profound aid possible from the outside. In a Pancha Sama cure the five (Sanskrit: "pancha") principles of Samarina, Samaya, Sambodhana, Sambhojana and Samshodhana are applied in an individually coordinated combination, creating a balance, a profound harmonisation and coordination (Sanskrit: "sama") in body, mind and soul.

We previously encountered Samarina and Samaya in connection with Ritam Samation. Samarina is the first part of it, the rebooting of the mind, and Samaya the second part, in which the toxins and waste products released are eliminated from the body and the physiology is restructured. Ritam Samation is, in fact, an integral part of a Pancha Sama cure, helping to cleanse and reorient the mind in a Samation routine precisely attuned to the patient and the continuation of the cure.

Sambodhana comes from the Sanskrit word for "insight" and "knowledge" and constitutes the main element of external support utilised in the cure. For this purpose, the six-handed, or sometimes even ten-handed, synchronised massages of Sambodha Ritam are performed at least once a day, likewise precisely geared to the course of treatment. It is the task of Sambodha Ritam to retransmit to the entire body – to every single cell – the correct information about its function in harmony with the whole. To this end, special pressure and stroking techniques are used by the practitioners in a specific order synchronically on the various parts of the body. In this way, all the cells are firstly reawakened directly or indirectly through the activation of particular reflex points and then stimulated in their functions by coordinating impulses. It is actually the case that a major percentage of our body's cells are not only undersupplied and underused due to our years of incorrect behaviour but are in fact lying in a "coma" – unconscious because of a lack of nutrients and stimulation. Because many deposits of waste substances are mobilised by Sambodha Ritam, thus making the supply routes available again, and the cells receive direct impulses, they awake to new life and, in turn, make themselves felt in the body – and the mind – again through their activity. That is why Sambodha

Ritam involves a concretely perceptible awakening on all levels, which continues for a long time even after a single session of treatment. This impact is further intensified in a Pancha Sama cure by the coordinated sequence of several treatment sessions and additionally supported by the systematic activation of special circulatory and metabolic mechanisms. In this work the therapists/ use special Sambodha Manas to harmonise and integrate their own thinking and feeling, thus also exerting beneficial influences on the patient from this level.

The next principle Sambhojana is the principle of nutrition, namely on all levels from the feelings and the senses to breathing and diet. Here, the basic laws of food consumption and food combination, which we talked about in the previous chapters, are precisely applied. In this respect, the foundation is joy and fulfilment always and everywhere, which are the goals of the entire process and the structure of the cure. In special cases, going without food completely, i.e. therapeutic fasting, may also be part of Sambhojana. In this way, our new-found friend, hunger, is used under the intensive supervision of the cure manager to carry out profound cleansing and clearing work in the body, which would otherwise only be possible over very long periods of time, if at all. Not for nothing is correctly practised therapeutic fasting also called an operation without a scalpel, for in a state of absolute abstention from food the body gets its nutrients from within, making use of everything that is not necessary for its functioning. And in precise terms, that is metabolic waste, foreign bodies, misguided macromolecules or confused body cells which impede its sound functioning in its normal state. Otherwise, Sambhojana provides the patient on all levels with the information they need for their recovery in the various stages of the cure.

Finally, Samshodhana, the principle of purgation, is another central feature of the cure, which also determines its course the most. For any new cleansing is only sensible when the old toxins and waste substances have been eliminated from the body. The purgation mainly takes place over the gut, kidneys and skin and is systematically supported by special massages, cleansing techniques, systematic sweating and dynamic exercise and also elements of Sambhojana. Finally, Samaya ensures that everything takes place lightly and gently, both on the physical and emotional levels.

You can now really imagine – and you actually experience it like that in the concrete situation – how such a cure gradually awakens all the cells and bodily systems from their dull comatose state and, just as in spring, they feel a fresh breeze of new activity, new vitality and new hope. In its laborious, daily struggle with the poor and inadequate supply of nutrients, only providing increasingly useless substances, every cell suddenly concretely feels relief, giving it a breathing space. More and more molecules exactly suited to its metabolic function arrive, also bringing joy and lightness with them, which dissolve the previous paralysing depression like swathes of mist in the morning sun. At the same time come regular impulses, movements, and reflex signals that shake the old encrusted deposits, allowing more and more air for deep breathing. This new mood spreads like wildfire through the whole body, everything comes alive, blossoms, sprouts, reaches out and stretches. A zest for life holds sway again, where previously only dismal staleness had prevailed, and every cell does its bit to support the large-scale cleansing. In this way, the heaps of rubbish vanish, the view is clearer, the horizon broader and a new lust for life can be felt everywhere. Digestion becomes easier, as the gut has been purged and, at the same time, much lighter food follows. The circulation revives, as the blood is thinner and, at the same time, the supply channels permit a more fluid transport with regular dynamic exercise bringing additional vitality. The immune system works at full steam as there is a lot to be disposed of. But, in return, the regular major alarm after meals is no longer necessary and as the external defence mechanisms are at last being reinforced, an enormous relief is overall foreseeable. The musculoskeletal system feels a new lightness coming up in it, as there are fewer problems with lubricating everything and altogether much more energy is available. Thus, a wave of joy spreads over the whole body and happiness hormones whir about like butterflies.

All this naturally also has its effect on the top management, which, in turn, gains new energy and insights through a different daily routine and regular deep relaxation. Gone are the times when every little coordinating task proceeded sluggishly. Now everything happens so easily and zippily that you really want more. The long-due clearing up in the basement provides additional relief. And the highlight of the day is the half-hour in the morning and evening when the mind is at last allowed to do what it likes, where it is relieved of all its obligations for a short time. What it can experience then! It lives from that for the whole of the rest of the day. The matrix it dives down into during this time provides it with a lot of interesting information, so many answers to questions it had been asking itself its whole life long, and so many impulses as to how it can accomplish its daily tasks better and more meaningfully. It is a true treasure trove! For this it is worth restructuring everything a little so as to have even more leisure time for more extended excursions. It actually should have thought of it much sooner! But somehow it had always been too narrow-minded. But that is now over – once and for all.

The soul is very content with this new development. It has an almost forgotten feeling of happiness, as the essential things in life are now important again. For the mind seems to be waking up at last and recollecting and the body is also now beginning to function in the way it had always longed for. At last, it is clearing away the heavy, oppressive hormones, which had so often taken its breathing air, beginning instead to live the lightness and agility the mind so badly needs to help it with its excursions to other spheres. What had it got the other two for after all! It had almost given up hope of them getting anywhere in this life. But that now seems to be a thing of the past, and it will also do everything possible for things to continue in this direction – on which point it is in complete agreement with the mind and body.

And that is it! Knowledge is emerging. During the Pancha Sama cure, the patient has had such a profound positive experience on all levels that they do not want to return to their previous state anymore. Now they no longer only have the information about what health really is but have experienced and felt it – they know it. And that is the basis for the patient not having any more difficulties in staying on the new course and pursuing it further – without coercion, sacrifice or lack. On the contrary, anyone who has once sniffed the ocean breeze - even if only for a brief moment - will not stop until they have reached the ocean and are able to refresh themselves in its cooling waves. Only in this way is real change possible – through information coupled with experience. Anything else remains on the level of the intellect or stuck somewhere inbetween so that you will stumble over one sausage stand after another for all eternity – till the penny simply drops one day.

Such a transformation of information into knowledge effects far more than just an improvement in physical symptoms. Naturally headaches and migraines disappear, naturally blood pressure, circulation, weight and digestion become normal, naturally varicose veins, cellulitis, asthma and many other complaints improve, but, above all, a profound transformation takes place on all levels of the personality. Everything – feelings, behaviour, physical reactions – changes. To a certain extent, a new program element is added to our operating system. That was also the way in which Jesus of Nazareth healed. He healed with the word, thus giving people information but at the same time enabling them to have such strong experiences due to his personality that the information immediately became knowledge and their entire physiology functioned accordingly. But this meant that it was not only healing on a physical level but at the same time a profound reprogramming of the mind and a release of the soul. There could no longer be talk of faith in God with the people concerned. It had become knowledge – real, genuine knowledge or Veda.

What does that mean for us here and today? It means that information is important but it has to be implemented without fail. For otherwise it cannot be transformed into knowledge – or exposed as wrong. Any implementation is, in fact at the same time, the perfect way to check the information and, in the end, only our own personal experience can show if something is correct or not. The intellect can, of course, do the preparatory work for this. For when it discovers inconsistencies or even logical contradictions, it immediately lets founded doubts arise about the correctness of the information.

But information which appears coherent in itself can also be wrong. In this very connection, there is a clear and unfortunately also up-to-date example. Let's imagine a health system based on the principle that everything in nature works correctly from the beginning, that our body thus possesses the optimal repair and regenerative mechanisms, which if a disease occurs at most have to be stimulated and promoted, whereupon it heals the disease itself if there is correct behaviour in harmony with the natural laws – even in serious cases. On the other hand, let's imagine a second health system, which assumes that the body, in fact, functions correctly in the normal case but in the case of disease is, however, not able to help itself, requiring external support at all cost. In the first system, a cleansing and regenerative cure would consist in bringing the patient's behaviour into harmony with the natural laws as optimally as possible and otherwise enhancing the body's own functions to their maximum through external measures. In the second system, the measures would, however, consist in reducing the body's own mechanisms to zero, if possible, and instead carrying out the cleansing by means of systematic external interventions.

At first glance, both systems appear sensible and plausible, although they are totally opposed. So let's have a look at the practical implementation of each of them. The treatment in the first system is the Pancha Sama cure, which we have just described in detail, and the treatment in the second system is the Pancha Karma cure in conventional Ayurveda, as is practised, above all, in India but also increasingly here in the Western world. In such a Pancha Karma cure, the digestive fire in the stomach and gut is initially reduced to a minimum during the first few days, by providing no or only very light food and with increasing amounts of saturated fat – mostly ghee – being drunk every morning on an empty stomach. After that, large quantities of oil, which was denatured beforehand by heating it to a high temperature, are introduced into the body via the skin with gentle stroking. According to the theory, the saturated fat now to be found in the body then releases the toxins and in the next step these are transported with systematic sweating cures to the gut, from where the therapists finally remove them with medical enemas. These measures are additionally supported by artificially induced vomiting or purging and also by sniffing in special oils or herbal blends through the nose.

After this description, anyone who possesses basic physiological knowledge will already know that this cannot work and will even backfire. However, all others think they first have to try it out. For however strange and unfamiliar most of the things sound, many people still think they must somehow be effective, as this method, after all, originates from a very old tradition and so everybody cannot have been mistaken. However, this is the very point where their thinking is wrong. For if everyone thinks in this way – and perhaps that was really the case up to now! – these drastic treatment practices will continue to be practised forever, causing harm to many more credulous people.

The fact is that the practice of the Pancha Karma,which we have just described, constitutes a considerable health risk, which even those responsible warn about "in weak patients". For it unfortunately only too often happens that the digestive fire does not begin to function again for a long time after such a cure, with the gut also suffering considerable injuries. On the other hand, the positive effects are mostly minor – apart from chance spontaneous self-cleansing by the body, triggered by the extreme irritation. Not for nothing is it recommended to carry out a Pancha Karma cure several times a year.

In connection with the subject of "information", we can imagine what it means for the body when, for instance, it is given pure ghee on an empty stomach, deliberately outsmarting its natural nausea, or when oils, salt, honey or vegetable stock are inserted into the colon, where they have no reason to be by nature. At any rate, health will not be achieved by this, let alone the true health we are aiming for. At the same time, however, it will also become clear to us from this example that a great deal of valuable information has got lost in conventional Ayurveda, which is still based on the same natural laws as AyurVeda Ritam. However, the difference consists in conventional Ayurveda being based on old writings, which it takes to be authoritative truth only because they are old. Yet, these texts were not written down until many centuries after the era of Vedic high culture and that, in turn, by people who did not rely on their own consciousness but alone on the teachings of their master. For example, does it not already make one suspicious when the Samas, the body's basic modes of action, are described as "Doshas" – Sanskrit: "mistake, health disorder" and bear the names "Vata" – Sanskrit: "wind, air" –, "Pitta" – Sanskrit: "gall" – and "Kapha" – Sanskrit: "mucous, phlegm"? What kind of information is released and disseminated on the vibrational level, where it actually ought to be a question of health and the highest form of existence!

Equally shattering is the balance of a comparison with Western medicine, which we might view here as a third system, which no longer assumes that the body can function faultlessly alone, even in its normal state. According to this theory, the body even has some functionless or useless organs, such as the tonsils or the appendix, and beyond a certain age absolutely everything goes wrong unless supporting chemicals are introduced from outside.

But we do not want to detain ourselves with these systems of obvious ignorance, for there we will certainly not find any clues in our search for true health. However, the question arises more and more clearly as to where we can search at all, if even the oldest traditions contain such errors and modern scientists are still groping with their knowledge in the most profound darkness. Why don't we simply do what Samuk Deda did? He had exactly this question and was faced with exactly the same problem. But instead of searching outside, he went inside into the depths of his consciousness, where the mind also strives to go in Ritam Samation and where it comes into contact with the matrix, the vibrational blueprint of the whole of creation. It is the initial implementation of basic knowledge – Veda -, the construction plan of the universe. Like a mould for the whole of existence, it contains all information, all data and all laws. There he found what he was looking for and from there AyurVeda Ritam stems – avoiding all faulty written records, erroneous traditions or biased scientific investigation - straight from the source.

That sounds very grandiose, like enlightening inspiration with heavenly spherical sounds and visions of all possible angels, Devas and good spirits. But it was not and is not like that. I myself once asked Samuk this question and he replied in his simple, natural way:

"You know, most people have high-flown esoteric ideas when it is a matter of higher or original knowledge. But all animals and plants have this knowledge in themselves and it is the most normal thing in the world. Only we humans think a lot about it because we have lost it because of our wrong behaviour. But once we behave correctly again, as the natural laws stipulate, the knowledge also comes back – just as normally and naturally as with every daisy or every ant. I did nothing else but simply bet on the horse of natural laws. In doing this, my body and mind experienced a deep cleansing and I more and more often had the experience that I was able to answer questions I actually asked myself as well. When I checked, I was shown unmistakably that the answers were correct. But where did these answers come from if I myself hadn't known anything about them previously? Quite obviously from the level of the matrix. Through the regular practice of Samation and the continual, ongoing cleansing, my mind again and again had access to this level, on which all the answers are to be found – even to questions we have not asked yet at all! In the end, it doesn't matter where our mind has got the information from. The important thing is to implement it, check it, thus transforming it into knowledge – or reject it. It's quite simple. Everyone can do it."

That is the point which is important for us. "Everyone can do it" – if they behave correctly. So let's get going!

In this book we have obtained all the basic information to be able to answer the crucial question as to what is important for us in this life, what has priority. We have also seen what importance information has and that, in fact, everything in nature is information. But it has also become clear that information is far from being everything. It has to be implemented, lived and become knowledge. For only then does it differ from dusty books or lifeless computer discs and acquires real importance for our life, for existence. Knowledge is everything and without knowledge everything is nothing. That is shown by the examples of the Hunza tribe and Thomas Parr, whom we spoke about in this book. For in the end they became victims of their ignorance. But what might they – and Linus Pauling as well – have become if they had had perfect knowledge!? So let's set out and get the knowledge for ourselves. The basic information is already available to us thanks to AyurVeda Ritam. We now first of all have to let it become knowledge by implementing and living it. For it constitutes the first few rungs of the ladder. We will then ourselves experience and thereby also prove everything that will develop out of it on the higher rungs. So don't let us dream and theorise about quantum leaps, life expectancy, special capabilities or true health but let us live them! For if Samuk Deda found access to the level of the matrix, we can do it too – every single one of us. To do it, however, we have to behave accordingly – if we want to.

Anyone who is still hesitating or is even disappointed that this book – like all the books in the world – cannot convey more than information, should remember Thomas, the young student in chapter 6. He did not let himself be led astray by his disappointment and gave Samation a chance with himself. Neither did he dither around with his diet for a long time but immediately implemented the information from every single paragraph of his book, even before he had finished reading it. He thus benefited, even though he recognised one thing or another as not so good and stopped doing them again. At any rate, today he has come much nearer to the knowledge of life, gaining new insights daily – of dimensions of whose existence he had had no inkling at that time. For when access to the matrix is free, things really start happening!

References

- The Influence of Cooking Food on the Blood Formula of Man, Paul Kouchakoff, First International Congress of Microbiology, Paris, 1930
- Nouvelles lois de ḃalimentation humaine basées sur la leucocytose digestive, Paul Kouchakoff, Mémoires de la Société vaudoise des sciences naturelles, Lausanne, 1937
- Nutrition and National Health, Sir Robert McCarrison, Faber and Faber, 1953
- Youth in Old Age, Dr. Alexander Leaf, John Launois, McGraw-Hill, 1975
- Diet and Exercise as a Total Therapeutic Regimen for the Rehabilitation of Patients with Severe Peripheral Vascular Disease, Longevity Research Institute, 52nd Annual Session of the Congress of Rehabilitation Medicine, Atlanta, 1975
- Regression of lesions in canine atherosclerosis, M. Bevans, J. D. Davidson, F. E. Kendall, Arch. Path. 51:228, 1951
- Relative Failure of Saturated Fat in the Diet to Produce Atherosclerosis in the Rabbit, William E. Connor, Jay J. Rohwedder, Mark L Armstrong, Circ. Res. Vol. XX, June 1967, p. 658
- Regression of Coronary Atheromatosis in Rhesus Monkeys, Mark L. Armstrong, Emory D. Warner, William E. Connor, Circ. Res. Vol. XXVII, July 1970, p.59
- Heart Victims on 10-Mile Walks in New Program, The Sun, 10. Dez. 1975
- The Stress of Life, Dr. Hans Selye, McGraw-Hill, 1978
- Aerobics, Kenneth H. Cooper, Evans & Co, 1978
- How to Live Longer and Feel Better, Linus Pauling, W. H. Freeman & Company, 1986
- Wege auf Wasser und Feuer. Ultraman, Klaus Haetzel, Econ, 1989
- Strength increases from the motor program: Comparison of training with maximal voluntary and imagined muscle contractions, Guang Yue, KJ Cole, Journal of Neurophysiology, 67, 1992
- Laufende Promis: Im Rathaus sitzt ein Iron Man, Michael Heinrich, Laufzeit 2/94

- Surgeon General's Report on Physical Activity and Health, U. S. Department of Health and Human Services, Centers for Disease Control and Prevention, 1996
- El Cerebro Consciente, Jacobo Grinberg-Zylberbaum, Editorial Trillas, 1979
- El Espacio y la Conciencia, Jacobo Grinberg-Zylberbaum, Editorial Trillas, 1981
- Looking for Doctor Grinberg, Sam Quinones, New Age Journal, July/August 1997
- Vorsicht Geschmack, Udo Pollmer, u. a., Rowohlt, 2000
- Health and Light, John N. Ott, Ariel Press, 2000
- Mental gymnastics increase bicep strength, New Scientist, Nov. 2001

Internet:

- USDA National Nutrient Database,
  http://www.nal.usda.gov/fnic/foodcomp/search/
- http://www.veg.org
- http://www.veggie.org
- http://www.vegsoc.org

Around the Subject

The Author

After his studies of mathematics, physics and other natural sciences in Germany and the USA, Dr. Hoffmann did a PhD in applied mathematics and has since been occupying himself intensively with concrete applications of natural laws in human life.

On this basis together with Samuk Deda he developed the basic universal health system AyurVeda Ritam and the original astrological system JyotirVeda Ritam.

Further Reading

- Hoffmann, Dr. Thomas: AyurVeda Ritam – Gesundheit aus erster Hand, Julia White Publishing, 2003, ISBN 3-934402-11-9

- Hoffmann, Dr. Thomas: Das Licht im Sturm, Julia White Publishing, 2003, ISBN 3-934402-01-1

www.ingramcontent.com/pod-product-compliance
Lightning Source LLC
Chambersburg PA
CBHW031516270326
41930CB00006B/418